THE PEANUT ALLERGY ANSWER BOOK

THIRD EDITION

Michael C. Young, M.D.

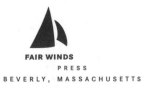

FAIR WINDS
PRESS
BEVERLY, MASSACHUSETTS

First published in the USA in 2013 by
Fair Winds Press, a member of
Quayside Publishing Group
100 Cummings Center
Suite 406-L
Beverly, MA 01915-6101
www.fairwindspress.com

First edition 2001
Second edition 2006

17 16 15 14 13   1 2 3 4 5

ISBN: 978-1-59233-567-1
Digital edition published in 2013
eISBN: 978-1-61058-914-7

Library of Congress Cataloging-in-Publication Data available

Cover design: Kathie Alexander
Book design: tabula rasa graphic design

Printed and bound in the United States

*The information in this book is for educational
purposes only. It is not intended to replace the advice of
a physician or medical practitioner. Please see your health
care provider before beginning any new health program.*

THE
PEANUT
ALLERGY
ANSWER
BOOK

THIRD EDITION

This book is dedicated to my loving wife and daughter and to my father, who have provided me with their encouragement, inspiration, and love.

I also dedicate this book to the loving memory of my mother, who gave up her career as a young physician to raise my sister and me and inspired us to the call of medicine and learning.

And to all who have food allergies, and to the dedicated people who work hard to make this world a safer place for them, you inspire me and humble me, I dedicate this book to you.

CONTENTS

CHAPTER 3
WHAT YOU NEED TO KNOW ABOUT ANAPHYLAXIS

CHAPTER 7
PREVENTION OF PEANUT AND OTHER FOOD ALLERGIES

CHAPTER 8
THE FUTURE OF PEANUT ALLERGY TREATMENT

ACKNOWLEDGMENTS

One of the true pleasures of practicing the specialty of allergy is having patients who are genuinely interested in finding out the causes and triggers of their problems rather than just treatments and cures. Allergy patients are interested in learning about their problems and how to prevent them. Over the years, I have had the privilege of caring for many patients and their families. I have learned much from all of them, and they are directly responsible for this book.

I would like to extend my deepest gratitude to all of my patients. In particular, I would like to thank Christopher Smith, at the time a peanut-allergic toddler, and his mother, Lisa Lavieri, who looked for a book on peanut allergy and was unable to find one. She discussed this with her sister, Holly Schmidt, who was then publisher of Fair Winds Press. Holly subsequently contacted me to write this book. I owe Chris, his mom, and his Aunt Holly special thanks for the genesis of *The Peanut Allergy Answer Book*. Holly was highly influential in my early days as an author, greatly improved my writing, and helped shape this book in its early stages of development. For that, I will be always grateful. Particularly satisfying to me is that since the publication of the first edition of this book, Christopher has outgrown his peanut allergy and is now a healthy 16-year-old!

I gratefully acknowledge and thank all my teachers and colleagues, especially my mentors, during my allergy fellowship training at Boston Children's Hospital, doctors Raif Geha, Donald Leung, Frank Twarog, and Martin Broff, who gave me the opportunity to join his practice. I also thank my many colleagues for reviewing the first edition of this book and giving helpful comments and suggestions: Doctors S. Allan Bock, Martin D. Broff, Raif S. Geha, Donald Leung, James Rosen, Hugh Sampson, John S. Saryan, Lynda Schneider, Albert L. Sheffer, Frank Twarog, and Dale Umetsu.

I have a special word of thanks to Anne Muñoz-Furlong, founder of the Food Allergy & Anaphylaxis Network (FAAN)—she is the model of what a dedicated parent can do. She single-handedly revolutionized the field of food allergy by forming the most important organization in the field of food allergy, serving patients, the medical community, and the general public. If my patients provided me with purpose in writing this book, Anne gave me inspiration. Anne has retired and FAAN has merged with the Food Allergy Initiative to become Food Allergy Research & Education (FARE), but their mission and good work continues. I also thank Terry Furlong and Chris Weiss, formerly of FAAN, who contributed to the section on airlines and peanut allergy. I thank Cara Connors, my current editor at Fair Winds Press, who provided invaluable insights and assistance for the third edition of this book. Thanks to her, this edition is the best yet!

I am delighted that for this third edition, the foreword is written by celebrity chef and author Ming Tsai. In addition to being a renowned chef and owner of two popular Massachusetts restaurants, Blue Ginger and Blue Dragon, having his own TV show (*Simply Ming*), and authoring five books, Ming has tirelessly advocated for the cause of food allergy and food-allergic people. His son had multiple food allergies since infancy and early on, Ming wanted to do something about the tremendous difficulties facing food-allergic children and their families. Ming started by making Blue Ginger one of the first food allergy–safe and –friendly restaurants, and then extended his efforts to being an advocate and spokesman for the field of food allergy on a local and national level. He helped in the passing of a Massachusetts law in 2010, requiring the education and training of restaurant staff in food allergies, the first law of its kind in the United States. I am honored with Ming's involvement with this book and also happy to report his son is now 13 and has resolved his food allergies!

Finally, I thank my family, especially my wife Karen and my daughter Liane, whose understanding and love provide me with the inspiration for all that I do.

FOREWORD

In 1999, about the time my son David was around six months old, my wife, Polly, and I noticed he had a rash that wouldn't go away. Turns out it was eczema, which, in infants, is an indicator of food allergies. After testing, he was diagnosed with seven of the eight major allergens: soy, wheat, dairy, shellfish, peanut, tree nut, and fish. Imagine that, the son of a chef being born with major, life-threatening food allergies? Now that's a twist of fate. We soon joined the world of parents trying to navigate the confusing landscape of children's allergy information and responsibility.

You could say David kick-started my passion and advocacy for allergy awareness. I, in a sense, found my calling. Today, I am proud to be part of many collective efforts taking action and providing assistance to today's allergy-challenged families.

I am a huge fan of the author. Dr. Young and I first met at Children's Hospital when he was David's doctor. Our paths have also crossed many times since then. Besides being a top allergy and immunology specialist, he has spearheaded some amazing programs (with Food Allergy Research & Education [FARE] and the children's show, *Arthur*, on PBS) to help families learn together on how to live with allergies. He helps them understand how to be vigilant, to recognize potentially problematic foods, and to eat more safely.

This third edition of *The Peanut Allergy Answer Book* is another example of Dr. Young's incredible work. Since it was first launched in 2001, *The Peanut Allergy Answer Book* has been a key resource for anyone seeking answers surrounding peanuts as allergens. And what's even more remarkable, by publishing the updated editions, Dr. Young helps maintain the relevancy and accuracy of the available information. This third edition has newly expanded sections in research and treatments to help families be more informed in these critical areas.

Despite the vast amount of data, the beauty of Dr. Young's book is the simplicity in how it's put together. There are easy-to-understand chapter titles along with key content formatted as frequently asked questions (FAQs). This gives readers the flexibility to either quickly locate their immediate topic or more casually scan to identify areas where they, in time, will want to explore.

I am honored to know Dr. Young and so appreciative of all his work. As we witness the increasing number of people with food allergies, especially children, resources like *The Peanut Allergy Answer Book* are not just a convenience, but also a necessity for today's families to be healthy and safe.

—Ming Tsai
FARE Ambassador Who Cares
Chef/Owner Blue Ginger and Blue Dragon

PREFACE
TO THE THIRD EDITION

In the twelve years since the initial publication of *The Peanut Allergy Answer Book*, there have been huge changes. Even as the numbers of peanut-allergic children continue to increase, the field of peanut allergy and anaphylaxis has seen great advances in research and treatment and has become the most exciting and active area in the specialty of allergy and immunology.

In my research for the third edition of this book, I reviewed more than 200 new scientific publications on peanut allergy alone, including studies on the underlying mechanisms of how allergic reactions occur, promising new methods of treatment, management and prevention of peanut allergy and anaphylaxis, new diagnostic tests, new information on the continuing increase in the prevalence of this allergy, and new insights into why the peanut allergy epidemic is uniquely a feature of Westernized countries.

In the past ten years, as the prevalence of peanut allergy has tripled in young children, public awareness of the societal impact of peanut allergy has greatly increased, with more and more peanut-allergic infants and toddlers entering daycare, preschool, and school. This has led to the publication of guidelines for schools in the management of food allergies and anaphylaxis, the enactment of the Food Allergen Labeling and Consumer Protection Act of 2006 and the Food Allergy & Anaphylaxis Management Act of 2011. There is proposed legislation for having stock epinephrine in schools and national restaurant guidelines for food-allergic consumers.

Many of these strides have been due to the huge effort of the Food Allergy & Anaphylaxis Network (FAAN), advocating for all food-allergic patients, educating schools, communities, the public, and not only funding scientific and clinical research, including a global symposium on anaphylaxis, but actively conducting research studies, and supporting local, state, and national legislative efforts to make the world a safer place for people with food allergies. FAAN has changed, too, merging in November 2012 with the Food Allergy Initiative, a private foundation formed by concerned parents and families to fund food allergy research, to become Food Allergy Research & Education (FARE).

Despite all these accomplishments, despite increased scientific knowledge and understanding, and despite schools and communities working harder to protect and safeguard peanut-allergic children, anaphylactic reactions continue to occur, and tragically, fatal food reactions have not decreased. The role of information and education in this area of medicine has never been more important. Our work is not finished!

I wrote this book to bring together all the available information necessary to understand and manage this important medical problem in an easy-to-read question-and-answer format. Returning readers of the previous editions will find the original material has been extensively updated and revised, with more than 50 percent new information, all still in the same user-friendly format. The bibliography in Appendix D has been updated with many new references and studies so you can go to the original sources for more information. I encourage you to use the table of contents for the specific questions you have. You do not have to read this book in order; many readers refer to the specific questions as they occur over time or just browse through the questions that interest them. There is also a lot of useful information for people allergic to other foods besides peanuts. Much of the general information can be applied to you as well.

I wish to thank the many readers of the first and second editions for their very helpful comments and suggestions; you are the inspiration for this new edition. As knowledge and progress in peanut allergy continues in the coming years, I will continue to update and revise *The Peanut Allergy Answer Book* for future editions.

INTRODUCTION

Since the original publication of this book in 2001, the prevalence of peanut allergy has tripled. Where I might have routinely seen four or five patients a week with peanut allergy just five years ago, I now often see more than five or six a day, for the same problem. Most of the people with peanut allergy I saw fifteen or more years ago were adults; now my peanut-allergic patients, particularly those with new peanut allergies, are exclusively very young children and infants.

The number of people, especially young children with life-threatening allergic reactions, has also dramatically increased. There has been heightened interest in peanut allergy, especially with the recent attention focused on banning peanuts from schools and airlines. The commonplace occurrence of peanut and peanut products in our daily lives presents an enormous challenge for peanut-allergic people and their families. More than 5 billion pounds of peanuts are produced a year in the United States alone, more than any other country. According to the U.S. Peanut Council, 11 pounds of peanut products are ingested annually by the average American. About 55 percent of peanuts are consumed in the form of peanut butter and the remainder are consumed as table nuts and in baked goods and candies. Peanuts and peanut products, especially peanut butter, are an inexpensive and convenient food source and have become very popular as snacks and quick meals, often substituting for regular full meals in many busy households. As a result of this increased exposure, emergency medical care and hospitalizations for allergic reactions continue to increase. Peanut allergy is unfortunately a potentially life-threatening allergy and for most children a lifelong problem that is usually not outgrown.

The most commonly asked question I encounter is why is there so much more peanut allergy now than just a generation ago? When I first wrote this book in 2000, it was believed that infants and very young children were more susceptible to food sensitization due to their immature immune systems. For that reason, the advice to families at that time was to avoid feeding peanuts to children before age 3. However, instead of decreasing, peanut allergy has tripled in prevalence since 2000! As you will see in this updated edition, studies now indicate that delaying the introduction of peanuts in the child's diet may actually increase the risk of peanut allergy! There is a paradigm shift in our whole understanding of peanut allergy.

When I was first approached to write this book in 2000, I was surprised to learn that there were no available books specifically on the subject of peanut allergy. From the large numbers of patients I follow in my private practice in Massachusetts and in the allergy program at Boston Children's Hospital, I knew there was a definite need for a comprehensive book on this subject. This book is written for the increasing number of people with peanut allergies and their families. It addresses the many issues they face, from knowing which foods contain peanut and peanut products, to understanding how to deal with peanut exposures in daycare, schools, and airlines, to performing emergency planning in the event of a life-threatening allergic attack.

In my practice and in my reading of the medical and consumer literature, I found people asking the same questions. This book is written and organized in a question-and-answer format to address those commonly asked questions. I have tried to make medical terms easy to understand. Use the glossary in the back of the book for new terms. Many of these new words are boldfaced in the text. From reading this book, you will learn how to successfully prevent and manage this problem and thus will not have to live in constant fear of life-threatening exposures. You will learn all you need to know about peanuts and allergies and will be able to design strategies to cope with this allergy. I have my many patients to thank for the inspiration for these questions and for the concept of this book.

CHAPTER 1

ALLERGIES IN A NUTSHELL

What are food allergies?

Matthew is a six-month-old baby who has been breast-fed since birth. At two months of age, his mother introduced rice cereal into his diet with no problems. Subsequently, she gave him oatmeal and applesauce, and at five months of age, he had egg for the first time. He developed a very itchy, dry, and scaly rash on his face, which, over the course of several weeks, worsened to involve the creases of his arms, the backs of his knees, and his neck and ears. His pediatrician diagnosed "baby eczema" and prescribed a moisturizer and hydrocortisone cream. The rash improved, but did not resolve. It seemed to worsen after he ate, but there was no consistent pattern. His mother brought him to my office and allergy tests showed he was allergic to milk, soy, egg white, wheat, and peanut. His rash significantly improved with the elimination of these foods from his diet.

The symptoms of food allergy in children typically involve the skin. Hives are common, particularly on areas of contact such as the mouth, lips, and face. In severe cases, these areas can become swollen and intensely itchy. When the skin becomes chronically inflamed, the rashes take the form of eczema, a very itchy, dry, scaly eruption that often begins in early infancy. Typical areas of skin involvement are the face, arms, and legs, particularly the creases, knees, elbows, neck, and behind the ears. Gastrointestinal symptoms are also common, ranging from nausea, vomiting, and diarrhea to acute severe abdominal pain and colic. More subtle reactions can take the form of failure to eat and gain weight. Respiratory symptoms, such as wheezing, nasal congestion, and mucous secretion, are less common chronically but can be severe when they occur. Some people with asthma have food allergy, and their asthma can be triggered by the ingestion of the foods they are sensitized to.

Conversely, some people with food allergy who do not have asthma can experience an asthma-like reaction when they eat the foods they're allergic to. When these people are studied, they often have an asthmatic tendency, although their baseline lung function will usually be normal. What this means is that, although they do not have the diagnosis of asthma, they may be prone to chest symptoms such as chronic cough or wheezing with common colds, physical activity, and exercise. Finally, anaphylaxis, a life-threatening systemic allergic reaction, can occur. It is rare, but is, of course, the most dangerous of all allergic reactions and what we all work to prevent and avoid.

Food allergy is more common in children than in adults. It has been estimated that 6 to 8 percent of infants younger than age two are allergic to food, and approximately 1.5 percent of adults have food allergy. The common food allergens in children are milk, eggs, soy, wheat, peanuts, nuts, and seafood. Of these, milk, eggs, and peanuts cause 80 percent of all food allergies in children. In adults, the common food allergens are tree nuts, peanut, fish, and shellfish, which cause 85 percent of allergic reactions. A 2010 survey in the United States suggests that 2.1 percent of children are allergic to peanuts and tree nuts, compared with 1.2 percent cited in the previous edition of this book. Sensitivity to many foods, especially milk, eggs, and soy, tends to resolve with age, whereas allergy to peanuts and tree nuts often begins in infancy but fails to improve with age. For reasons that are still unclear, peanut allergy is associated with fatal anaphylaxis more than any other food.

Food allergies usually occur in individuals who also have other manifestations of allergic disease such as hay fever, asthma, and eczema. People with these allergic disorders have a greater tendency to develop sensitivities to food. Because allergies in general tend to be inherited, family members are often allergic as well, although not necessarily with the same allergies. Although allergies to specific foods are not inherited per se, the tendency to be allergic to food in general is genetic. Some recent studies now suggest the possibility of genetic transmission of peanut allergy.

How are food allergies related to the immune system?

Richard is a 43-year-old man who had milk allergy as a child and was affected by eczema and chronic diarrhea. After going on a dairy-free diet, he eventually outgrew these symptoms and was able to consume milk products by the time he entered school. He had no further allergy problems until he developed hay fever and asthma at age thirteen. These symptoms remain unchanged and are usually worse in the spring when the trees pollinate; he also has hives and wheezing when he is near cats and dogs. He has a two-year-old son with chronic eczema and recurrent ear infections who recently developed hives after ingesting peanut butter.

When people commonly think of allergies, they think of symptoms such as sneezing, itchy, watery eyes, and stuffy noses that occur when they get hay fever in the spring and fall. Some other people wheeze and have trouble breathing from asthma attacks when they exercise or when they "feel allergic." Still others become deathly ill when they are stung by bees and yellow jackets. How do all these different problems relate to the person who is unable to eat certain foods, such as peanuts or shellfish, and who breaks out in hives, experiences swelling of the throat, or has abdominal pain and diarrhea? These reactions are all results of the body's immune system reacting in an inappropriate way to what should be innocent and innocuous things in our daily lives. That is what an allergy is. To understand how this happens, we need to learn a little bit about how our immune system works and how this can cause us to develop allergies to different things. We will learn the definition of a few key words such as allergen, IgE, T and B white blood cells, mast cells, and histamine.

The immune system is responsible for protecting the human body from infection and invasion from bacteria, viruses, and other harmful agents by its ability to distinguish "self" from "nonself." Substances identified as foreign or "nonself" are attacked by cells of the immune system and destroyed or rendered inactive. The immune system in allergic people is different from that of nonallergic individuals in that it identifies innocuous and benign things, such as food, pollen, animal dander, and medications, as harmful to the body and targets them for an immune response. This response is a very potent inflammatory reaction that results from the production of a special protein called **IgE antibody**, which recognizes a specific allergic agent (**allergen**) in the same way that other antibodies (such as IgG, IgM, and IgA) recognize and fight bacteria and viruses. This recognition is very specific because a given IgE antibody is unique to one and only one allergen. So, peanut-**specific IgE (sIgE)** will recognize only peanut, and cat-specific IgE will recognize only cat dander. This is the reason why some people are allergic to certain things but not to others. Which things a person is allergic to are determined by which specific types of IgE antibodies he or she has, so that people allergic to peanuts will react to peanuts only and not to cat dander unless they also have cat-specific IgE.

The process by which the immune system initiates an allergic reaction to food begins with its recognition of the food allergen. Foods are composed of proteins, carbohydrates (sugars and starches), fats, minerals, and water. The allergenic portion of food is only the protein, and it is the food proteins that trigger immune recognition by white blood cells in the immune system called T cells. These T cells can then activate other white blood cells called B cells, to make the IgE protein specific for the food allergen such as peanut or egg. This IgE antibody circulates in our bloodstream throughout our whole body and finds its way to various tissues and organs such as the skin, gastrointestinal tract, lungs, nose, and eyes. On reaching these areas, the IgE attaches to cells called **mast cells**, which are located in these organs and tissues. Once the allergen-specific IgE is attached to the mast cells, you become sensitized to that particular allergen.

Mast cells are important in allergies because they make the chemical **histamine** as well as other chemical **mediators**. Histamine is what directly causes the many symptoms of allergies such as itching, hives, stuffy nose, and wheezing. We use **antihistamines** because they are medications that block the actions of histamine, thereby blocking allergic symptoms. When the sensitized tissues come in contact with the allergen—through eating or breathing, for example—the allergen attaches to the tissues by means of the allergen-specific IgE mast cell complex. This attachment causes the mast cell to release large amounts of histamine and other similar chemical mediators into the blood. Histamine circulates through the blood and to surrounding tissues and subsequently binds to these tissues by means of histamine receptors. Antihistamines work by inhibiting the binding of histamine to these tissue receptors.

Histamine binding results in many tissue reactions and changes, including congestion, swelling, mucous secretion, itching, and sneezing. In the lungs, constriction of air passages results in shortness of breath, wheezing, and difficulty breathing. In the gastrointestinal tract, vomiting, diarrhea, and abdominal cramping result. In the skin, itching, swelling, hives, and eczema result.

In the most severe reaction, the cardiovascular system is affected, resulting in a drop in blood pressure, shock, and potentially death.

This potentially fatal reaction is called **anaphylaxis**. Anaphylaxis can involve more than one organ system, e.g., the sufferer can experience both hives and wheezing, or both itchy throat and vomiting. The allergens that are the most common causes of life-threatening anaphylaxis are the allergens that are absorbed into the body internally such as food, medications, insect stings, and, in certain instances, latex rubber. The most potent food allergens are peanuts and tree nuts, fish, and shellfish. Of these, peanut is most frequently associated with near-fatal and fatal reactions. I will discuss the treatment and prevention of anaphylaxis in later chapters.

How do you know whether you have a food allergy?

I have always loved all kinds of seafood, especially shellfish. I was attending a meeting of allergists and had just returned to my hotel room following a delicious buffet luncheon where quite a bit of seafood had been served and where, following my appetite, I had indulged, especially in the lobster and crab dishes. I noticed that my entire chest and abdomen were suddenly intensely itchy and hot. I noted on my watch that approximately 30 minutes had gone by since I had finished lunch. I took off my shirt and was surprised to see myself covered in large red hives. I looked in the mirror and saw that my entire body was bright red. I also felt my heart racing and a tightness in my throat. "This must be what early anaphylaxis feels like!" I thought. I had never felt this way before. Luckily, I had some antihistamine samples I had received earlier in the meeting. I took two tablets and tried not to panic. After all, I was at an meeting full of allergists! Surely, someone must have epinephrine!

Fortunately, the itching and hives started to recede, and after a long hour, I felt much better but quite sleepy from the side effects of the antihistamine. I missed the rest of the meeting that day. The following morning, my allergist colleagues asked me where I was. Apparently, I had missed an interesting lecture on food allergies! Later that week, when I returned to work, I skin-tested myself with our panel of common allergenic foods. I had a positive skin test to crabmeat and was negative to everything else. In the 6 years since that incident, I have meticulously avoided crabmeat but have eaten other shellfish and seafood with no problems. I recently repeated the skin test to crabmeat, and it was negative. Subsequently, I have resumed eating crabmeat with no problems.

Food allergies are usually recognized initially by the person or person's family. Allergic symptoms such as itching, rashes such as hives or eczema, abdominal pain, nausea, vomiting, diarrhea, and breathing difficulty are all common symptoms of food allergy. When the symptoms occur in a consistent and recognizable pattern, following the ingestion of a specific food, it then becomes obvious that food allergy may be the cause of the various symptoms the person is experiencing. For example, ingestion of peanuts can result in the immediate eruption of hives, swelling, and difficulty breathing. This is not subtle, and you can make the diagnosis easily.

When the symptoms are chronic and inconsistent, it may be less clear whether the cause is a specific food or several foods, or perhaps not even a food at all. Seeing an allergy specialist to assist in the diagnosis or to document suspected food allergy may be very helpful. The allergist can sort through confusing symptoms and make deductions and conclusions on the basis of your history. He can also perform allergy testing to confirm the presence of specific food allergies. The allergy specialist has the special training to do this.

How do I choose an allergist?

An allergist specializes in the diagnosis and treatment of allergic diseases and asthma. Allergists complete an additional six years of specialty training after receiving their medical degree. An allergist needs to complete training and pass the board examinations in either internal medicine or pediatrics before being allowed to take the allergy board examination. Allergy specialty training consists of three additional years of training in allergy and immunology in fellowship programs, during which the doctor will learn about how to diagnose and treat hay fever, asthma, eczema, and food, drug, and insect allergies in children and adults. Choosing a board-certified allergist will ensure that your doctor has completed the required allergy and immunology training and passed the examination for the allergy specialty. Your primary care physician is the best person to contact regarding a referral to the best local allergist for you. Your primary care physician would have an established relationship with that doctor and know his or her particular style and expertise with allergy patients. Your doctor may know the allergy specialist's particular interests, which may include food allergies. The American Academy of Allergy, Asthma and Immunology (www.AAAAI.org) and the American College of Allergy, Asthma and Immunology (www.ACAAI.org) are national organizations of allergy specialists and can give you the names of all the allergists in your local area. Other organizations that can be helpful with referrals to allergists are the local chapters of the American Lung Association and the Allergy and Asthma Foundation of America, as well as your local medical society.

As with selecting any adviser, whether a doctor, lawyer, accountant, or broker, you want, first of all, to meet the allergist and talk to him or her to determine whether there is compatibility, compassion, and trust. A good doctor will above all *listen* to you and allow you to speak freely about your problem and your concerns regarding it. The art of good medicine is to be able to take a thorough history from the patient, and you can tell a lot about the doctor's knowledge from his or her questions. Frequently, good questions can help guide you to think about the problem better, and ultimately you might be able to come up with answers yourself. If you are a parent, observe the doctor's ability to relate to your child and whether a rapport develops. Never underestimate the ability of a child to describe his or her observations. A good doctor experienced with children can elicit this history effectively, even from small children. Go to the doctor appointment with a specific list of questions and concerns. Things always seem more confused and hectic during the appointment, so having something concrete to refer to will make the process much smoother and easier.

What information does your doctor need to diagnose food allergies?

Doctor, I have food allergies!
Please describe your symptoms.
I have nausea and pain in my stomach every time I eat.
Have you noticed which foods cause these symptoms?
I can't really tell, it seems that all meals will do it.
How soon after you eat do you feel nauseous and stomach pain?
Sometimes, it's during the meal, and at other times, it's a few hours afterward.
Do you have any other symptoms along with the nausea and pain, such as itching, hives, swelling, or difficulty breathing or swallowing?
Yes, but I get those all the time, not just with eating!

Food allergy symptoms can be very difficult to sort through, and often the symptoms are vague in nature, making it difficult for you and your doctor to diagnose. The key to solving this puzzle is a history carefully taken by an allergist or a physician with experience in dealing with food allergies. The physician will take a detailed history of your symptoms, paying special attention to the sequence of reactions and correlating the timing of your symptoms with the specific foods eaten. Severely allergic people usually experience their reactions within 30 to 60 minutes after they eat. Delayed symptoms sometimes do occur, and this makes it harder to determine which food is the cause of the reaction. In this situation, it is the consistency and pattern of responses that can help clarify what is going on.

How a Food Diary Can Help

One of the most useful tools in the diagnosis of food allergy, for both the doctor and patient, is a carefully kept journal in which you record your exact symptoms (e.g., itching, hives, nausea, abdominal pain, trouble breathing, etc), the timing of the first symptoms in relation to meals and eating, and, most importantly, a complete list of everything eaten.

Ideally, this list should include not only all foods and beverages, but also the ingredient lists of all processed foods consumed. The reason for this is that, as we'll learn later in this book, there are many hidden foods and ingredients contained in products that are not always obvious. Artificial flavorings, dyes, and preservatives can also cause allergic reactions in some people. Recording how much of the food you eat is important, especially the smallest amount that will cause a reaction. The most recent reaction as well as the number of times that a reaction has occurred with each food is also helpful.

Review of this information can give great insight into whether or not specific foods are responsible for specific symptoms. Often, hidden sources of exposure, such as cross-contamination, can be deduced from a carefully recorded food diary. Food diaries can also be helpful in assessing chronic conditions, such as eczema or chronic gastroenteritis, in which acute exacerbations and attacks may be rare.

What are the different kinds of allergy tests and how do they work?

The suspicion of food allergy can be verified by performing allergy tests on the person. Allergy testing is usually performed by an allergy specialist. The allergist has specialized training and certification in the treatment of allergic and immunologic diseases, including the diagnosis and management of food allergies. The allergist is the specialist best able to interpret the results of allergy testing. Determination of specific food allergies can be done by either **skin prick tests** and/or blood tests called **specific IgE tests** (sIgE) (formerly referred to as RAST tests and ImmunoCAP tests).

In skin testing, a very diluted extract of the actual food is used. The allergenic extract material is processed and purified by commercial laboratories. A drop of the liquid extract is placed on the skin; a plastic or metal point is then used to prick the skin just enough for the extract material to penetrate the skin but without actually breaking the skin. If the person is allergic to the extract material, his or her skin mast cells will already be sensitized to it and the person will have a histamine mediated reaction. The histamine will cause a small hive where the skin was pricked in the skin test.

When performing skin tests, your allergist will also administer a positive control with histamine to demonstrate that the skin is capable of reacting. The normal skin response of all people is to have a reaction to histamine with some itching and redness and a small hive. In some situations, however, the skin response to histamine is blocked or diminished, and the skin would not respond to any allergen testing either. The most common situation in which the histamine response is absent occurs when you have taken antihistamine medication before the skin tests. You should stop taking antihistamine medications 5 to 7 days prior to skin tests, otherwise your histamine response, as well as your response to any potential allergen tests, may be blocked.

You doctor will also administer a negative control with saline (a salt water solution) to control for the possibility of false positive skin tests caused by certain sensitive skin conditions. Skin tests can be read in 20 minutes and are inexpensive and minimally uncomfortable, with minor itching being the main effect. In children younger than two years, the skin may not always be reactive, and false negative skin tests may result. Some doctors suggest that following a negative skin test, the test should be repeated using a fresh sample of the actual food because there may be loss of activity or potency in the manufacturing process of the extract material.

Studies show that the size of skin tests to peanuts, milk, egg, and fish can predict whether a patient will pass or fail a food challenge to those foods. So, if the skin test is a certain size or larger, we already know the patient will react to that food and a food challenge would not be necessary.

Repeat skin testing as a child grows older may predict whether he or she is outgrowing that food allergy if the skin test size consistently decreases with age.

What is a specific IgE test?

Blood tests used to diagnose allergies were referred to as the RAST test, which stands for "radioallergosorbent" test. The original technique involved radioactive reagents but most laboratories currently use nonradioactive "tracers" that rely on color changes in the reagents. "RAST test" has persisted as a generic term for allergy blood tests in the same way that we refer to photocopies as Xeroxes or cellophane tape as Scotch tape.

Currently, the medical community favors the use of the term "specific IgE test," which is precise and does not indicate a specific method or manufacturer. The blood test works by detecting the presence of allergen-specific IgE in your blood. Blood is drawn from your arm and sent to a laboratory for processing. This involves adding your blood to the allergen, which has been attached to a paper disc, plastic plate, or cellulose matrix. Following a timed interval, this mixture is washed and a "tracer" anti-IgE antibody is added to detect the binding of your IgE to the allergen. The amount of allergen-specific IgE contained in your blood sample can be calculated from this result. How high, or positive, the specific IgE test is reflects how much antibody you have to that specific allergen. Although the specific IgE test is slightly less sensitive than skin prick tests, it can be useful in people who are unable to stop antihistamine therapy, people who have extensive skin disease, or people in whom there is a significant risk of anaphylaxis from the skin testing. The main problem with specific IgE tests is that the results can vary considerably from laboratory to laboratory because of differences in laboratory technique and procedure as well as quality control.

Currently, the most accurate and reliable specific IgE blood test is the ImmunoCAP system. This system has been studied in comparison to other specific IgE blood test methods and has been shown to more accurately measure the degree of allergy for four foods in particular—peanut, milk, egg, and fish. In food challenge studies, the ImmunoCAP blood test is the system that more accurately predicts the outcomes of the challenges. The ImmunoCAP levels are measured in units called kU/L and range from < 0.35 to > 100. The levels of allergen-specific IgE measured by the ImmunoCAP system correlate with how active your symptoms are and if these levels decline, it may indicate that you are losing the allergy. It may be a better way of following food allergies, because skin tests can remain positive, even when clinical activity lessens as a child "outgrows" the food allergy. I recommend repeating the specific IgE levels for food allergy every year or two in children, particularly if you are interested in the following the course of the food allergy over time. Most, but not all, hospital and commercial laboratories now use the ImmunoCAP system for measuring allergy blood tests. If your test results are not in the kU/L units, the test was not done by the ImmunoCAP method. You can have your doctor check to see whether your local lab uses this method.

Can allergy tests predict the severity of a reaction?

No. Neither skin prick tests nor specific IgE blood tests will predict the severity of reaction to any given exposure to peanut. The skin test and specific IgE test do indicate the activity of the allergy. The larger the skin test diameter and the higher the specific IgE level, the more "active" the allergy is, the more likely a reaction will occur on exposure, and the less likely you will be able to outgrow or resolve your peanut allergy.

Hugh Sampson, M.D., director of the Jaffe Food Allergy Institute in New York, found that if your peanut-specific IgE level was 15 kU/L or greater, you would have a 95 percent chance of reacting to peanut on a challenge. However, even though the likelihood of a reaction will be high, the actual reaction symptoms can be mild, moderate, severe, or even fatal and are not predictable by testing. The reaction to any given exposure is dependent on many different factors such as the amount of exposure, the route of exposure (ingestion vs. skin contact, e.g.), and your health status at the time of exposure (e.g., whether you have active allergy and asthma symptoms). The adjectives often designated by each blood level, such as "mild" or "severe," are misleading and serve no purpose. They are completely arbitrary and because specific IgE levels do not predict the severity of reactions, these adjectives are meaningless and should be ignored.

In the future, there may become available a blood test that is able to predict the severity of clinical reactions as well as how likely the allergy might be outgrown. In 2004, Wayne Shreffler, N.D. and his colleagues published a new laboratory test called a microarray immunoassay (MIA), which measures the amount of IgE binding to **epitopes**, regions of the peanut protein that attach to the patient's IgE. The structure of the peanut protein's epitopes has been found to correlate with the severity of reactions as well as how permanent the allergy can be. The amount of binding of a patient's peanut-specific IgE to certain epitopes of the peanut protein and the total amount of binding in this MIA blood test correlated with severe reactions and the likelihood of outgrowing the peanut allergy. This MIA test is still under investigation and not yet available, but it holds much promise for the future management of peanut allergy.

How accurate are allergy tests?

The accuracy of an allergy test is determined by how often it correctly predicts a reaction will occur when you are exposed to that allergen. There is always a range of accuracy for any test. When a test is positive but you have no problems being exposed to that allergen, the test is said to be a "false positive." If, on the other hand, a test is negative but you get reactions from that allergen, the test is "falsely negative." For food allergies, tests can be falsely positive more than 50 percent of the time! On the other hand, the rate of false-negative results is much lower, particularly with skin tests. False-positive allergy results are often caused by similarities in proteins that may be found in foods belonging to the same food family. For example, because peanuts and soy both belong to the legume family, there are similarities in the protein structures of both plants and these similarities cause the tests for both peanut and soy to turn positive. Peanut-allergic patients who do not have problems with eating soy often have positive test results for both foods even though actual clinical reactions only occur with peanut. In fact, 90 percent of peanut-allergic patients can eat soy.

What are component-resolved diagnostic tests and are they more accurate than skin tests and specific IgE tests?

A commercially available blood test for food allergies called "component-resolved diagnostic tests (CRD)" has become available. These blood tests measure individual food proteins. As said previously, food proteins are the allergenic "components" of foods that trigger the immune system to make specific IgE antibodies that cause allergic reactions. (See "How are food allergies related to the immune system?" on p. 21.) Every food contains numerous proteins, some or all of which can be allergenic. For example, milk contains casein and whey proteins and egg contains ovalbumin and ovomucoid, among others. Peanut contains multiple component proteins called Ara h 1, Ara h 2, Ara h 3, up to Ara h 11. "Ara" is short for *arachia*, which is the Latin name for peanut. When peanut-specific IgE levels are measured, the total amount of peanut-specific IgE is measured, which is the sum of Ara h 1-specific IgE up to Ara h 11-specific IgE. Studies have shown that patients with a history of allergic reactions to peanuts have high levels of specific IgE for Ara h 1, Ara h 2, and Ara h 3 but their levels of Ara h 5, Ara h 8, and Ara h 9-specific IgE do not seem to correlate with a history of peanut allergy. These other peanut proteins share similarities to proteins found in pollen and other plants and legumes and are not associated with allergic reactions to peanuts.

Component-resolved diagnostic testing (CRD) measures each specific component protein, for example, milk casein-specific IgE. CRD testing will more accurately predict a person's likelihood of reacting to peanuts if their CRD testing is positive for Ara h 1 and Ara h 2–specific IgE, which are closely associated with a history of peanut reactions. This test is particularly useful for patients diagnosed with peanut allergy from screening allergy tests, either positive skin tests or specific IgE tests, who have never eaten peanut. As discussed previously, having a positive skin test or blood test does not necessarily mean that an allergic reaction will occur. The test could be falsely positive. In this situation, the CRD test would helpful in predicting whether that person would actually have an allergic reaction from eating peanuts.

There are some studies indicating that severe anaphylactic reactions to peanut correlate with levels of Ara h 2–specific IgE, but studies have not yet been performed using the commercially available CRD test to predict anaphylaxis. At the present time, I do not recommend using the CRD test as an assessment of the severity of peanut allergy. I do think the CRD test is useful in patients where the diagnosis of peanut allergy is uncertain because of the lack of history or lack of clarity in the patient's skin tests and blood tests.

If I can eat peanuts without any problems, even though my peanut allergy tests are positive, should I stop eating them?

If you are already eating peanuts and nuts and are not having any problems, you are not allergic to them and there is no need to do allergy testing for peanut and nuts. If you have already been tested for peanut allergy, despite having no problems eating peanuts, and the tests come back positive, you can disregard these false positive results and continue eating peanuts. Allergy testing done on a screening basis, without any preceding history of definite reactions to that food, can result in false positive tests that are clinically irrelevant and actually cause much confusion and unnecessary elimination of foods that have been well tolerated. Random allergy testing of the general population without regard to any clinical history generally results in positive tests 5 to 6 percent of the time. In ordering allergy tests, doctors must base their test selection on your clinical history. I do not generally order screening panels of foods except for patients with a gastrointestinal disorder called eosinophilic esophagitis, an inflammatory disease of the esophagus. In many patients with this disorder, food allergies can cause the inflammation, and elimination of those foods can improve or even resolve this disease.

What is a food challenge?

Ultimately, the only way to know whether a food will cause a reaction is to actually eat it and see what happens. If eating the food causes symptoms consistently, that food is a problem. If elimination of the food eliminates the symptoms you are having, that food would certainly be suspect.

Using an elimination-and-challenge procedure is a practical way for testing your suspicions regarding any suspect foods that may be causing you problems. A food that, when eliminated from your diet, results in improvement, and when eaten again causes your symptoms to recur, is a problem food that should be avoided. This elimination-and-challenge procedure can be used to test suspect food allergies in your diet that you think are the cause of your symptoms. However, if the symptoms are severe allergic symptoms such as swelling or breathing and swallowing difficulties, this procedure is too dangerous to do on your own—especially for foods commonly associated with anaphylaxis such as peanuts, nuts, and seafood. Instead, it is best to undergo testing and possible challenge procedures under your doctor's supervision in his or her office, clinic, or hospital so that your safety is never compromised.

An oral food challenge consists of giving a very small amount of the food and then increasing the amount every 15 to 20 minutes and observing for any signs of an allergic reaction. The procedure is stopped at the first sign of any allergic symptom. If there are no symptoms, the amount of food administered is increased up to an amount comparable to a real-life portion, such as a tablespoon. To eliminate any biases on the part of the patient or the doctor, the challenge can be "single-blinded" for the patient or "double-blinded" for both the patient and the doctor.

The definitive method of diagnosing food allergy is the **double-blind placebo-controlled food challenge (DBPCFC)**. It is useful to understand the DBPCFC method because it is referred to frequently in the food allergy literature. The DBPCFC is a functional test that seeks to reproduce the patient's actual symptoms by direct challenge. Therefore, it can be useful in the diagnosis of non-IgE mediated food reactions such as lactose intolerance, as well as classic food allergies. The DBPCFC method eliminates the possibility of patient bias and investigator bias by "blinding" both sides so that neither the patient nor the physician knows whether the actual food or **placebo** (a dummy sample that contains no food protein) is being given. There are many symptoms and reactions that can be mistaken for food-allergic reactions, so it is important to be able to objectively assess and separate these reactions from true allergic reactions.

To illustrate this concept, Keith Rix, a psychiatrist at Leeds University, England, studied twenty-three patients with a history of food reactions. All patients were able to consistently identify the foods that triggered their reactions. However, when the foods were administered blindly through a tube directly into the stomach, the only four individuals who had any symptoms were the four who had convincing histories of anaphylaxis. Five of the nineteen nonresponders walked out of the study when it became obvious they were not reproducing their allergic symptoms with the food they claimed to be allergic to.

The placebo effect is another important factor that can complicate any medical study. A placebo is the so-called "sugar pill" or "dummy pill" that contains no active ingredient, whether it be medication or food. Its purpose in a challenge test or medical study is to measure the person's response to what he or she *believes* to be the real food or medication. Placebos can cause many different symptoms such as cough, headache, itching, wheezing, and high blood pressure. Studies show that people can actually be addicted to placebos. The effectiveness of placebos has been shown to be 35 percent, which is higher than many medicines on the market! Therefore, any scientifically sound study has to account for the placebo effect by using a control group of patients who are given a placebo in a "blinded" fashion, so they do not know whether they are being given the study food or a placebo. The food or placebo is given in a capsule that is tasteless, giving no clue to its contents. The code telling what each capsule contains is sealed until the end of the study. Once the study with both food and placebo capsules is completed, the seal on the code is broken, and the results can be tabulated. If the person's symptoms are reproduced with the food and not with the placebo using the DBPCFC method, the diagnosis of the food-specific allergy can be made.

The danger of any challenge method is the possibility of inducing anaphylaxis in the allergic individual. Obviously, challenges should be done only in a medical facility capable of treating anaphylaxis. If the actual amount of food that caused the reaction is known, graded smaller concentrations of the food can be used sequentially in the challenge procedure, building up to the actual amount that was originally ingested. This increases the safety of the procedure. From a scientific point of view, the DBPCFC is considered the "gold standard" for the diagnosis of food allergy. Although the DBPCFC can be performed in your allergist's office, it is usually performed in a hospital setting.

For most cases of peanut allergy, the history of an immediate reaction to ingestion or contact with peanut, confirmed with a positive skin prick test or specific IgE test, is sufficient for diagnosis; a peanut challenge is seldom necessary to diagnose peanut allergy. In my practice, I usually order peanut challenges to see whether my patient has outgrown or resolved peanut allergy. This point is reached when the skin and blood tests indicate a low likelihood of a reaction.

What is the youngest age to undergo a food challenge?

The purpose of a food challenge is to see whether the suspect food will cause actual symptoms when ingested. At the first sign of a reaction, either observed by the patient or the doctor and nurse supervising the challenge, the procedure is stopped. The initial reactions many patients experience during challenges are often very subtle, such as mild discomfort in the throat, mouth, or lips. We rely on the patient to communicate these symptoms during the challenge so we know when to stop the challenge. By the time the doctor or nurse actually observes symptoms such as hives, swelling, or difficulty breathing, the reaction has already progressed to a more severe level and the patient might already be uncomfortable and require medications to reverse the reaction. A very young child is often incapable of communicating these symptoms. Mentally challenged patients and patients with communicative disorders also fall into this category. I generally consider doing food challenges in children starting at age 3 or 4, depending on their level of communication and understanding of the procedure.

What is an elimination diet?

Andrew is 3 years old and has had severe eczema since age 6 months. He was evaluated in my office, and skin tests showed allergies to milk and eggs. I recommended eliminating all milk and egg products from his diet. On his follow-up appointment, he still had significant eczema, although it was less extensive than before his diet. On close questioning, it appeared that he was still eating some baked goods at his grandmother's that were cooked with milk and eggs. Once these foods were eliminated, Andrew's eczema was much easier to control.

When you suspect food allergies, but are not entirely certain which foods are the cause, an elimination diet can be the answer. An elimination diet completely and strictly eliminates each suspect food for a certain time period. You should make the original list of suspect foods, from a careful analysis of your food and symptom diary and medical history. If the symptoms persist, despite a carefully done elimination diet, screening allergy tests such as skin prick tests or specific IgE tests might help narrow down the list or screen for foods that were not originally suspected.

Once you make a list of suspect foods, you and your physician can design an elimination diet. The diet has to be completely free from the suspect foods, including products containing and cooked with the foods, and all possible hidden sources of the foods. The greater the number of foods to be eliminated, the more difficult the elimination. Ideally, the elimination period should be 2 weeks. If your symptoms resolve during that period of elimination, you have found a possible cause. If the symptoms persist despite the elimination diet, it is unlikely that the suspect foods were relevant and you might then proceed to other possible foods. An elimination diet should only be done under a physician's supervision to avoid the possibility of any nutritional deficiencies.

If the elimination diet to select foods was unsuccessful in resolving the symptoms, the next step would be going on an **elemental diet**. Elemental diets are essentially allergen-free formulas that are nutritionally complete in proteins, fats, and carbohydrates. Examples of elemental infant formulas are Neocate and Elecare. Pregestimil, Alimentum, and Nutramigen are hypoallergenic formulas that do contain small protein fragments or peptides. For adults, Vivonex is available as well. An elemental diet is a rather extreme alternative but if it fails to resolve your symptoms, you can be reasonably sure you don't have a food allergy.

If the symptoms do resolve, the next step is to reproduce the symptoms by direct challenge. This is ideally done by DBPCFC, but an open challenge can be considered if the skin or specific IgE test is negative and the actual history is rather doubtful for allergy. In this situation, the risk for anaphylaxis is low and the challenge is fairly safe to perform in the office. Food challenges should never be done at home if there is even a remote chance of anaphylaxis or severe symptoms occurring.

The confirmed diagnosis of a food allergy is made when the

elimination of the offending food resolves the symptoms and when challenge with the offending food reproduces the symptoms.

Are there food reactions that aren't allergies?

Reactions to foods can occur by mechanisms other than allergic reactions. Food intolerance can occur in individuals whose digestive system is unable to digest and metabolize food, resulting in undigested or partially digested food, which can then lead to bacterial overgrowth, diarrhea, gas formation, and abdominal pain and cramping. Lactose intolerance is probably the most common example of this, occurring in 5 percent of the Caucasian population but in as much as 60 to 90 percent in African-Americans, Hispanics, and Asians. Because people with lactose intolerance are unable to digest lactose, the major sugar in milk, they often mistakenly believe that their intolerance of milk is actually a milk allergy. Although milk avoidance is the treatment plan for patients with lactose intolerance just as it is for milk-allergic patients, the mechanisms for their respective problems are very different.

Skin testing and specific IgE testing will detect only allergen-specific IgE, so these tests will not be helpful in the diagnosis of food intolerances and other types of adverse food reactions in which IgE is not involved. Skin tests and specific IgE tests performed on these individuals will be negative. Most children with milk allergy will outgrow the problem. Most people with lactose intolerance have it as a permanent condition. Many, however, are able to tolerate varying amounts of dairy products in their diet depending on the severity of their condition.

Another example of a non-IgE mediated food problem is celiac disease, in which gluten, a protein found in wheat, rye, and barley, triggers an inflammatory reaction in the small intestine resulting in symptoms of abdominal pain, bloating, diarrhea, and weight loss caused by failure of the small intestine to absorb nutrients. Patients with this disease need to avoid wheat, rye, barley, and other gluten-containing foods and additives. Because lactose intolerance and celiac disease are not allergic disorders, allergy testing for the milk and wheat proteins will be negative. These are disorders affecting the digestive tract so there is no risk of respiratory symptoms or anaphylaxis with these diseases.

CHAPTER 2

PEANUT ALLERGY 101

What is the historical background of peanut allergy?

Peanuts probably originated in eastern Bolivia and were cultivated for food at least as early as 2000 to 3000 B.C.E. The ancient Peruvians considered peanuts so important that they buried their dead with pots of peanuts to accompany them to the afterlife. Fifteenth-century Spanish explorers brought the peanut back to Europe and then to the Philippines and Indonesia. Their popularity spread to Vietnam and China by the 1700s and subsequently from China to Japan. The Portuguese brought the peanut to Africa in the 1500s, which later spread to India. The English and French were cultivating peanuts by the 1700s.

The American biochemist, inventor, botanist, and educator George Washington Carver (1860–1943) is given credit for developing the many modern uses of peanuts. He was interested in enriching the nutrition of minorities and the poor, and peanuts provide a highly nutritious and inexpensive source of easily digestible protein. Peanuts also are an excellent source of niacin (vitamin B_3), vitamin E, magnesium, chromium, and manganese. These nutrients are typically found in meats, whole grains, legumes, and vegetable oils. The peanut's versatility and ability to be prepared in so many forms, eaten whole as a vegetable, roasted and salted as a snack, crushed and ground as a spread or "butter," and incorporated into candy, baked goods, and other foods was ideal for Carver. It could also be used for cooking oil, which was extracted by pressure or solvents. Carver discovered more than 300 uses for the peanut, including the manufacturing of plastics, adhesives, bleaches, and linoleum.

In addition, the cultivation of peanuts and the manufacturing of peanut products were important sources of employment and remain so to the present. The United States, particularly the southern states, remains one of the world's largest producers of peanuts, along with China and India. Seven states account for approximately 98 percent of all peanuts grown in the United States: Georgia (38 percent), Texas (23 percent), Alabama (10 percent), North Carolina (9 percent), Florida (6 percent), Virginia (5 percent), and Oklahoma (5 percent). There are about 40,000 peanut farms in these peanut-producing regions. The contribution of peanuts to the U.S. economy is $4 billion a year.

Annual peanut consumption in the United States is nearly 1.7 billion pounds, or about 11 pounds per person, of which more than half is in the form of peanut butter. Peanut butter was invented in the 1800s and popularized by John Harvey Kellogg, who invented corn flakes. The first recipe for the peanut butter and jelly sandwich was published in 1901 and by the Depression era, the peanut butter sandwich was one of the most popular food items for children. Peanut butter has been a staple of the American diet since and is found in 75 percent of households.

What is the history of peanut allergy in medicine?

As early as the fourth century B.C.E., Hippocrates observed that milk could induce hives and gastric upset. Food allergy was first recognized as a clinical entity in 1921 by German physicians Otto Prausnitz and Heinz Kustner. The first definite reference to nut allergy in the medical literature was in 1920 by the noted hematologist Kenneth Blackfan, M.D. He observed a 10-year-old child with eczema that was "always intensified" after consuming nuts, eggs, and fish. "The eating of any of them was followed almost immediately by a burning sensation in the throat, vomiting, diarrhoea, oedema of the lips and ears, and urticaria."

There was no research in the field of peanut allergy until as recently as 1978, when S. Allan Bock, M.D., reported fourteen children with peanut allergy proven by direct challenge. In 1981, Steve Taylor, Ph.D., reported ten patients with peanut allergy who ingested encapsulated peanut oil without any allergic reactions, suggesting that peanut oil was not allergenic. In 1984, Hugh Sampson, M.D., and R. Albergo, M.D., showed that positive skin prick tests and RAST tests to peanut correlate 100 percent with positive challenge to peanut, establishing the usefulness of these allergy tests in the diagnosis of peanut allergy.

In 1988, John Yunginger, M.D., reported fatal anaphylaxis to food in seven patients, four of whom turned out to have peanut allergy. In 1992, Sampson reported thirteen patients with fatal and near-fatal food anaphylaxis, seven of whom had peanut allergy. Of the six patients with fatal anaphylaxis, four were allergic to peanuts. Both reports emphasized the great risk in delaying the administration of epinephrine to patients experiencing anaphylaxis.

In 1989, Bock and F. Dan Atkins, M.D., showed that peanut allergy in childhood usually persists into adulthood. In 1992, Donald Leung, M.D., and his colleagues reported three patients with peanut anaphylaxis successfully treated with immunotherapy to peanut extract. However, the rate of systemic reactions to the therapy was very high at 13 percent. In 2003, Leung, Sampson, and colleagues reported on the successful use of an anti-IgE vaccine in preventing anaphylaxis in peanut-allergic patients. By blocking all IgE in the body, this vaccine decreases all allergic reactions caused by IgE, such as peanut allergy. Patients who previously could tolerate only half a peanut before reacting could subsequently tolerate up to nine peanuts after the vaccinations.

Recent studies now show that 20 percent of peanut-allergic patients can outgrow their allergy by age 6. In 2009, a study was published showing the effectiveness of orally desensitizing patients with peanut allergy by administering small measured amounts of peanut.

Much current research has focused on the immunology and molecular biology of peanut allergy, characterizing the specific proteins causing IgE-mediated reactions. This research has led to successful gene sequencing and cloning of peanut protein. Using this information, several laboratories are working on potential vaccines for peanut allergy and other potential techniques for treatment, and biotechnology laboratories in the food industry are working on a nonallergenic peanut. If you are interested in learning more about the studies mentioned in this chapter or throughout the rest of the book, please see chapter 8 and Appendix D for specific references.

How common is peanut allergy?

Current estimates show that approximately 1.2 to 1.5 percent of children in the United States, Canada, and the United Kingdom are affected by peanut allergy. The prevalence of peanut allergy alone is 0.6 percent of the U.S. population. For children, the prevalence of peanut or tree nut allergy is 2.1 percent, compared to 1.2 percent in 2002 and 0.6 percent in 1997. For peanut allergy alone, the prevalence in children tripled from 0.4 percent in 1997 to 1.4 percent in 2008.

A British study showed that one in 200 four-year-olds have peanut allergy. One percent of all British preschool students are estimated to be affected. These infants and toddlers are particularly susceptible to peanut allergy; a recent study showed that peanut-allergic patients had their first allergic reaction at an average age of twenty-two months.

A 2003 Canadian study of 4,339 school children showed a 1.5 percent prevalence of peanut allergy, confirmed by allergy testing. A study of eighty-one children with a history of food allergies by Charles May, M.D., and Bock showed that 21 percent of these patients had peanut allergy by double-blind food challenges.

Comparing peanut allergy to other food allergies, 2.5 percent of newborn infants are allergic to cow's milk in the first year of life, and

15 percent retain this allergy into their second decade of life. Egg allergy occurs in 1.3 percent of children. Shellfish allergy occurs in approximately 0.5 percent of the population. Peanuts are by far the most common cause of food anaphylaxis.

Frequency of Food Allergies in Children and Adults

Food	Children	Adults
Milk	2.5 percent	No data available
Egg	1.3 percent	No data available
Peanut	1.2 percent	0.6 percent
Wheat	0.4 percent	No data available
Soy	0.4 percent	No data available
Tree nuts	1.1 percent	0.5 percent
Fish	0.1 percent	0.4 percent
Shellfish	0.1 percent	2 percent

Source: Scott H. Sicherer, M.D., Hugh A. Sampson, M.D., *Journal of Allergy and Clinical Immunology*, 2010; 125: S116–125.

Another study found that of 185 infants, 80 percent had been exposed to peanut products by age one and 100 percent had exposure by age two. Follow-up at age seven showed that 7 percent of high-risk children tested positive to peanut, and 4 percent had definite reactions to peanut by history or actual challenge. Sampson, a prominent investigator in field of food allergy and director of the Jaffe Food Allergy Institute at New York's Mt. Sinai School of Medicine, has observed a 95 percent increase in the number of allergic reactions to peanuts in both children and adults percent over the past 5 years. This increased prevalence of peanut allergy is consistent with the reports of allergists across the country as well as worldwide.

Why have peanut allergy and other allergic diseases increased so dramatically, particularly in young children?

The answer to this question is complex. There has certainly been an increase in all allergic diseases in young children, with a doubling in the numbers of children with asthma, environmental allergies, eczema, and all food allergies. The increase in peanut allergy probably parallels this general increase in all allergic diseases in children. The question that naturally follows is, "Why are all these allergic conditions so common in young children now compared to less than one generation ago?" There have been a number of theories to explain this increase. The theory that seems to have the most support from laboratory and clinical studies is the "hygiene hypothesis."

What is the hygiene hypothesis and how is it related to peanut allergy?

One of the initial studies leading to the hygiene hypothesis was the observation that before the Berlin Wall came down, East German children had much lower rates of asthma compared to West German children despite higher rates of air pollution, tobacco smoking, lower rates of childhood immunizations, and poorer socioeconomic status, and public health conditions. The more hygienic society seemed more allergic!

Multiple studies from Europe have found that children born and raised on farms and exposed to farm animals have lower rates of allergies and asthma compared to children raised in urban and suburban environments without any exposure to farm animals. These lower rates are associated with exposure to bacteria associated with the farm animals' fecal and waste products in the environment.

An interesting study from the University of Arizona compared asthma rates in children who grew up in daycare where respiratory illnesses, coughing, and wheezing were often the norm to rates in children who grew up in more sheltered environments and did not experience frequent respiratory illnesses. The asthma rates were surprisingly higher in children who did not grow up in daycare conditions, again showing that a more hygienic infancy period predisposed these babies to a more allergic outcome later in childhood. Subsequent laboratory studies in animals and humans suggest that the immune system in early infancy is primed to recognize and fight infections. In the absence of infections, the immune system is "reset" to target innocuous items in the child's diet and environment, resulting in abnormal reactions to harmless things such as food, pets, pollens, and dust mites. The exposures in the first few years of life seem to be critical in determining the child's subsequent development of allergies and asthma, or not having these problems.

Studies in Europe are now underway examining the possible use of probiotics, so-called good bacteria, in pregnancy and infancy as a way of turning off the "hygiene hypothesis switch." More recent work by Erika von Mutius, M.D., in Germany has indicated that there is less food sensitization in children raised on farms. This area of allergy and immunology is an active area of research that will yield very interesting and useful findings in the near future.

Why is peanut allergy more common in the United States, United Kingdom, and Australia compared to the rest of Europe, Asia, and the Middle East?

Prior to the 1980s, peanut allergy was a food allergy that was not increasing. However, reports of severe near-fatal and fatal anaphylactic reactions to foods were published with increasing frequency in the late 1980s and early 1990s. The most common foods associated with life-threatening reactions in these reports were peanuts, tree nuts, and shellfish.

Widespread concern regarding life-threatening food allergies prompted pediatricians in the United States and United Kingdom to recommend avoidance of peanuts, tree nuts, and seafood in children at risk for allergies, until they reached the age of three or older. Children with eczema and other allergic symptoms such as runny nose, wheezing, or with first-degree relatives with allergic problems were deemed to be at risk for food allergies. These dietary recommendations were made in the United Kingdom in 1998 and the United States in 2000. Assuming these recommendations were followed, you would think that food allergies would have leveled off or decreased after 2000. In fact, studies showed that peanut and tree nut allergy greatly increased in these countries whereas in countries where no dietary changes in children were made, peanut and nut allergy rates remained the same.

This observation raises the question of whether the deliberate avoidance of peanuts and nuts in children caused the increase in peanut and tree nut allergy. An interesting study published in 2008 by George DuToit, M.D., and colleagues from the United Kingdom examined this question. The study involved approximately 10,000 Jewish school children, 5,000 living in the United Kingdom and 5,000 in Israel. Peanut allergy occurred in 1.85 percent of the children living in the United Kingdom and only 0.17 percent in those living in Israel.

Because the study was on Jewish children only, genetic difference between the two groups was minimized. The only difference between the two groups of children was their diet: the British children had no peanut consumption in infancy between ages eight to fourteen months of age, whereas the Israeli children consumed more than 7 grams of peanut per month beginning between six to eight months old. These results seem to support the hypothesis that early introduction of peanut might actually reduce the risk of peanut allergy. In fact, when peanut consumption in different countries is examined, high rates of peanut consumption at an early age are associated with low rates of peanut allergy in children. This is true for countries in Asia, the Middle East, South America, and Africa. Interestingly, other studies that show early introduction associated with tolerance or delayed introduction associated with subsequent allergy, have been published for milk, egg, and wheat.

In China, the world's leader in peanut production, peanut consumption is comparable to this country and yet, peanut allergy is much less common. Peanut consumption in children begins early in infancy similar to the Middle East. Also, peanuts in the Chinese diet are usually boiled or fried compared to peanut butter and dry-roasted peanuts in the Western diet. Laboratory studies show that the higher processing temperatures used in manufacturing peanut butter and dry-roasted peanuts result in an increase in the allergenicity of the peanut proteins while the opposite is true when using lower cooking temperatures used in boiling or frying.

How does tolerance to foods develop?

The normal pathway for the infant and child is to be able to eat all foods. Allergies are the result of an abnormal immune response in a genetically prone individual who is exposed to the allergen and becomes sensitized (see chapter 1). The regulation of the immune response determines the pathway the individual will take—the allergic pathway or the normal pathway to "tolerance" with no allergies.

The T cells mentioned previously in chapter 1 are the white blood cells in the immune system that regulate immune responses, determining which responses become allergic reactions and which become "tolerance responses" where no allergic reactions occur. Whether allergy or tolerance occurs is determined by the amount of exposure, the route of the exposure (ingestion vs. skin contact), and the complicated interactions of one's genetic makeup and the environmental exposures of the hygiene hypothesis (infections, farm animals). How all this occurs is still quite speculative and not proven by studies.

It has not been established when the critical window of time in an infant's life is that determines how allergic that child will grow up to be, but it is most likely thought to be in the first six to twelve months of life. During this window of time, the regulatory T cells develop allergy or tolerance responses. It appears that ingestion of the food is required for tolerance to develop; without oral exposure to the food, the opportunity for tolerance could be lost. If subsequent exposure later in life occurs, such as through the skin, allergic responses can result. This is the hypothesis put forth by Gideon Lack, M.D., whose group did the studies comparing peanut allergy in the United Kingdom and Israel. Lack's group is currently conducting a study examining infant diet and the consequences of early feeding of allergenic foods such as peanuts vs. early avoidance, which, until recently, has been the recommended practice. (See chapter 7 for more details.)

What are the reasons for loss of food tolerance?

Approximately 20 percent of children with peanut allergy outgrow it by age six. Subsequent follow-up studies on these children showed that 8 percent had recurrence of their peanut allergy. The only risk factor observed for these relapsers was the continued avoidance of peanut and peanut products from their diet, despite having successfully resolved the allergy by passing food challenges. A variety of reasons explain their continued avoidance: they were so conditioned and used to their diet that change was difficult; they were still allergic to tree nuts and it was easier to continue avoiding all nuts; they didn't like the taste of peanut butter and peanuts; and their persistent anxiety about recurrence of their allergy prevented them from eating peanut.

The observation that continued avoidance of peanut resulted in loss of tolerance indicates that the ongoing ingestion and exposure to peanut is necessary to maintain tolerance. I advise my patients who have passed their food challenge to try and eat full servings of that food at least two to three times a week to maintain tolerance. If that is not achieved, I advise them to still keep their EpiPens available just in case.

There are also studies in the medical literature showing that food avoidance can lead to food allergy. Most of these studies are on children with eczema who underwent allergy tests to foods and who then eliminated those foods that were positive on testing to see whether their eczema would improve. Many of these children were eating these foods with no allergy symptoms at all, and none had ever had anaphylaxis. When prolonged elimination of the food was then followed by an accidental ingestion of that food, severe allergic reactions resulted, including anaphylaxis.

There is even a case report of a woman who developed milk allergy as a young child and avoided milk because of severe eczema. Her eczema eventually resolved but she developed severe milk allergy with anaphylactic reactions and unfortunately, had a fatal reaction at age 18 when she was accidentally exposed to a dairy product. It is important to strictly avoid all foods one is allergic to but avoidance of a food one has never had allergic reaction to could lead to loss of tolerance and increased risk of allergy to that avoided food.

Does early avoidance of peanut prevent or result in peanut allergy?

The answer to this question is presently unknown. Based on the information given previously:

1. that widespread observance of policies recommending strict avoidance of peanuts and nuts until age 3 not only did not prevent the epidemic of peanut allergy, but in the 8 to 10 years that followed those recommendations, peanut allergy tripled in prevalence,
2. that multiple studies show early introduction of milk, egg, wheat, and peanut result in less food allergy, whereas delayed introduction results in increased allergy,
3. that loss of tolerance to a previously tolerated food and subsequent allergy to that food can result from avoidance of that food,

it would appear that early avoidance of peanut in a child's life could increase the risk of allergy. If you ask your grandparents or great grandparents, they would say there was no peanut allergy in their childhood. All children then ate peanut butter and peanut products at an early age without restrictions. Peanut allergy became "epidemic" only after peanut butter was removed from children's diets in the 1990s and thereafter.

Lack has addressed this question in the LEAP (Learning Early About Peanut Allergy) Study, which began in 2007 and finished in 2013. He recruited 480 children ages four to ten months considered to be at risk for peanut allergy, having a history of egg allergy and eczema, and randomized half to eating peanut three times a week and the other half to strictly avoiding peanut. He is following these children until they reach the age of three years and then evaluating which group has more peanut allergy. When the results of this monumental study are published, we will finally have an evidence-based answer to this question!

Is peanut allergy hereditary?

Peter is a 31-year-old man with lifelong history of peanut and tree nut allergy. His mother and sister have food allergies but not to peanut. His wife has hay fever but no food allergies. She is pregnant with their first child, and they would like to know what their baby's chances of developing peanut allergy are.

It is well known that allergic diseases such as asthma, hay fever, and eczema cluster in families, and the individual often inherits one or more of the allergic diseases together. Food allergy is inherited, but whether allergies to specific foods such as peanut are inherited has not been extensively studied. Jonathan Hourihane, M.D., a prominent British peanut allergy researcher from the University of Southampton, examined fifty peanut-allergic children, their forty-nine mothers, forty-eight fathers, and forty-five siblings with questionnaires and skin prick tests. This study showed that all types of allergic diseases become more common in successive generations and occur more often in your maternal relatives than your paternal relatives. You are more likely to suffer from peanut allergy if one of your siblings has it than if one of your parents is allergic. The study showed that not only is peanut allergy inherited but also the tendency for all the other allergic diseases as well.

A study by Scott Sicherer, M.D., and his colleagues at Mount Sinai School of Medicine in New York published in 2000 examined seventy-four identical and fraternal twin pairs with peanut allergy recruited from the Food Allergy & Anaphylaxis Network. Among identical twins, 64 percent were peanut-allergic, whereas in fraternal twins, the concordance rate was 7 percent, which is the same as the concordance rate observed in non-twin siblings. These results strongly indicate the significant genetic influence on peanut allergy.

Should the sibling of a child with peanut allergy avoid peanuts?

Based on Sicherer's study on twins and non-twin siblings, the risk of peanut allergy in the sibling of a peanut-allergic child is 7 percent. I recommend that siblings of the peanut-allergic child be tested to see whether they are sensitized to peanut. If the skin tests or specific IgE tests are negative, they can start eating peanuts. On the other hand, if the tests are positive, that sibling should avoid peanut until he or she is old enough for a food challenge. Once the food challenge is passed, peanuts can then be safely introduced into the diet.

At how early an age can peanut sensitization occur?

Caitlin's mother first suspected Caitlin was allergic to peanuts when each time after eating peanut or peanut butter herself and then breast-feeding Caitlin, the baby became very irritable. When Caitlin was four weeks old, she developed an itchy red rash on her face, which also flared up after breast-feeding. At that point, her mother stopped eating peanut products. Caitlin was weaned completely from breast milk by six months of age. She was kept away from all peanut products until she was two years old. The very first time she was given peanut butter on a cracker she developed hives all over her body and had some wheezing as well. She was referred to me by the emergency room physician who treated her for that reaction.

Sensitization to peanut can occur very early in life. One theory is that this may be due to the high potency of the peanut allergens. One study showed that 80 percent of peanut-allergic individuals developed allergic symptoms on their first known exposure. A French study of newborn infants younger than eleven days and babies between age seventeen days and four months showed that 8 percent had positive skin tests to peanut. This certainly implies that sensitization occurred either shortly after birth or in the womb.

One study by Hourihane from the United Kingdom showed a correlation between the self-reported increased consumption of peanuts by pregnant and nursing mothers and a definite decrease in the age of onset of peanut allergy over the past 10 years. In other words, the more peanut products consumed by pregnant and nursing mothers, the younger the age at which their children developed their peanut allergies. Another more recent study by Sicherer and colleagues showed a correlation between the amount of peanut ingested by the mother during the third trimester of pregnancy and the risk of peanut sensitization in children with eczema and egg allergy.

However, other studies examining maternal diet and childhood peanut allergy did not show maternal peanut consumption increased peanut allergy. Although it is possible a pregnant mother's diet can affect her child's likelihood of developing food allergies, there is insufficient evidence from the current medical literature to make any recommendation for maternal diets as a strategy for preventing childhood food allergies.

Another potential route of sensitization is peanut oil–based vitamin preparations and infant formula. These items are a problem pri-

Should You Eat Peanuts While Breast-feeding?

Peanut proteins can be detected in breast milk for several hours after the mother has eaten peanuts. What this means is that an exclusively breast-fed baby can still be exposed to peanut protein and become sensitized to peanut through the mother. Babies with peanut allergies can develop allergic symptoms following nursing if the mother has recently eaten peanuts. Because a family history of allergic disorders such as hay fever, asthma, and eczema is a risk factor for the development of food allergy, it may be prudent for pregnant and nursing women with this family history to avoid allergenic foods such as peanut.

marily in Europe and are mentioned here to alert the traveler who might unknowingly make purchases of products that normally would not contain peanut oil in the United States. A report from France studied 122 children ages seven months to five years old. During the first two years of life, one group of children received vitamin D free from peanut oil, and two groups received vitamin D containing peanut oil. The two groups receiving vitamin D containing peanut oil had positive skin tests to peanut, while the group receiving peanut-oil-free vitamin D had significantly less sensitization on skin testing.

Most American brands of vitamins, such as Flintstones Supplements, One-A-Day, and Bugs Bunny vitamins, do not contain peanut oil. There is a report on the presence of allergenic peanut oil in milk formula in the British medical journal *The Lancet* from 1991, but to my knowledge, no American infant formulas contain peanut oil. Always be cautious when traveling abroad because of different practices in foreign countries. Topical creams and lotions can also contain peanut oils. Children with skin damaged from chronic inflammatory skin conditions, such as eczema, are probably most susceptible to sensitization from topical preparations. One of the few topical medications in the United States containing peanut oil is a steroid cream DermOtic, used for external ear infections. It is sold over the counter and does have a warning label for patients with peanut allergy. Most pharmaceutical-grade peanut oils contain no detectable levels of peanut protein, but it is certainly possible that the low levels of peanut protein that can cause sensitization are too low to be detectable by available technology.

What is it in peanuts that make them so allergenic?

John is a 25-year-old man with a lifelong history of peanut and tree nut allergies as well as egg, wheat, and soy allergies. He had an anaphylactic reaction at age thirteen when he accidentally was given some brownies that had nuts in them. He has been extremely careful about avoiding all nuts since then without any further problems. He has had mild hives after consuming egg, wheat, and soy products but never anaphylaxis.

———————

The answer lies in the part of the peanut that actually causes the allergy, the peanut proteins. Allergic reactions result from our body's immune responses to proteins; most food-allergic reactions are triggered by food proteins. In milk, the milk proteins are casein and the major whey proteins, lactalbumin and lactoglobulin. In egg white, they are ovalbumin and ovomucoid. In wheat, it is gluten and in shrimp, it is tropomyosin. The allergenic peanut proteins are the seed storage proteins vicilin, conglutin, and glycinin. By understanding the nature of these peanut proteins, scientists are beginning to unlock the mystery of why peanuts are among the most potent of all food allergens. The protein content of a peanut is 24.3 percent of the average weight of a peanut.

The allergenic proteins in peanuts are found in the cotyledon, or embryonic leaf, of the peanut seed plant. These proteins, like other food allergens, are glycoproteins, which are proteins that have sugars as part of their structure. Work from several laboratories has identified three major allergenic proteins from peanuts, called ara h 1, ara h 2, and ara h 3. Ara is derived from *arachia*, the Latin term for peanut. The genes for these allergens have been cloned and sequenced. ara h 1 belongs to the vicilin family of seed storage proteins, ara h 2 belongs to the conglutin family, and the most recently identified peanut allergen, ara h 3, belongs to the glycinin family. Ninety-five percent of peanut-allergic patients react to ara h 1 and ara h 2, while approximately 50 percent of peanut-allergic patients react to ara h 3. ara h 2 is the most potent allergenic protein of the three.

Additional minor proteins have been identified: ara h 5 through ara h 11. These minor proteins are clinically less important as peanut-allergic patients react to them less than 50 percent of the time. ara h 8 is structurally similar to birch tree pollen and ara h 5 is similar to proteins found in trees and grasses pollens. Sensitization to pollens commonly occurs in allergic individuals; falsely positive allergy tests to peanut can occur because of the similarities between the ara h 5 and ara h 8 peanut proteins and pollens.

Scientists have discovered some structural features of ara h proteins called epitopes. How strongly epitopes bind to IgE could explain why peanut proteins are such extremely allergenic proteins. With this information, researchers are now working on ways to alter the structure of this protein and hope that in doing so, a "hypoallergenic peanut" might be created that retains all the characteristics of a peanut except for causing allergic reactions. There is also research being conducted on creating vaccines to these peanut allergens.

Is the peanut a true nut?

Peanuts are vegetables, nuts, are fruits. Peanuts (botanical name *Arachia hypogea*) are actually members of the legume family, which includes lentils, soybeans, peas, black-eyed peas, lima beans, kidney beans, green beans, and garbanzo beans. Peanuts are native to South America and several varieties are grown in the United States. These include the Virginia, Spanish, and runner varieties. Peanuts grow in the ground unlike tree nuts, which grow on trees. The peanut plant is a bushy, flowering annual. After fertilization, the flower stalk elongates until its weight causes it to bend down and touch the ground. Continued growth of the stalk pushes the ovary into the ground, and the seeds grow, forming the familiar peanuts.

The botanical definition of a true nut is a hard, dry, closed one-seeded fruit. In general, the term "nut" can apply to any seed or dried fruit of a woody plant that does not belong to the legume family. The tree nuts commonly eaten and capable of causing allergies are walnuts, almonds, cashews, pecans, Brazil nuts, hazelnuts, Macadamia nuts, and pistachios. Almonds, pecans, and pistachios are the seeds of fruits. The fruit contains a pit that encloses the nut.

Almonds come in two types: sweet almond, which is the edible kind and bitter almonds, which are poisonous (although the oil can be extracted and is safe to use). Walnuts come in three varieties, black, English, and Persian. Pecans are related to hickory nuts and are covered by a leathery skin. Brazil nuts are the seed of large woody fruits. They include creamnut, chestnut of Para, and sapucaia or paradise nut. The cashew is the seed of a pearlike fruit that must be roasted to be palatable. The pistachio, sometimes known as the green almond, is also the seed of a drupe, like the almond and pecan. Piñon, or pine nuts, are the seeds of pines and are found in pine cones. Pignolia nuts are the seeds of the European pine and resemble pine nuts. The hazelnut, or filbert, is a true nut and the seed of a pearlike green fruit.

Other true nuts include acorns, beechnuts, which are primarily used for animal feed, and chestnuts. Macadamia nuts are also called Queensland, Australian Gympie, Bush, and Bopple nuts. The seed is contained in a fruit with a fleshy husk, and the thin shell of the seed is cracked to release the nut. Although many people are allergic to more than one nut, some people have just one solitary tree nut allergy.

Are there nuts that do not commonly cause allergies?
The coconut, not a true nut, is also the seed of a fruit but is generally not restricted from the diet of tree nut–allergic people. Other non-allergenic nuts found in other parts of the world are ginkgo nuts used in Chinese and Asian cooking, Pili or Javanese almonds, terminalia or wingnuts, found in the Orient, and Kola nuts. Water chestnuts, nutmeg, and mace are not nuts and do not need to be avoided by tree nut–allergic people. Shea nut butter is from the fruit of the Karite tree of Ghana, *butyrosperum parkii*. Shea nut butter is not actually from a nut, but is derived from pressing the whole fruit, which is much like an avocado. The slightly greenish butter from the shea nut has soothing, protective qualities and sunscreening properties, and can be found in many creams, lotions, and cosmetics. It does not need to be avoided by nut-allergic individuals.

Should you avoid all members of a food family if you are allergic to one food in that family?

Anne is 36 and recently married a Greek man who brings her to visit his family in Athens every summer. She has developed allergy symptoms to some Greek dishes experiencing hives, diarrhea, and on one occasion, wheezing. She thinks she is allergic to some of the spices such as parsley, dill, caraway, and anise. Her food skin tests were positive to celery and carrots, both members of the Umbelliferae family to which parsley, dill, caraway, anise, coriander, and fennel also belong. She tries to avoid all members of this food family but has trouble convincing her Greek mother-in-law of her allergy problem.

The prevailing thought at one time was that being allergic to one type of legume meant that you would cross-react to all members of the legume family regardless of previous exposure or history. Because peanuts are legumes, people allergic to peanuts were therefore advised to avoid not only peanuts but all members of the legume family, whether or not they had ever had a reaction to other legumes. To take this logic further, it was also a common belief that being allergic to one member of a food group automatically made you allergic to every food in that group. This theory was based on the work by John Vaughan, Ph.D., and Michael Black, Ph.D., in 1929, when they classified foods into botanically related food groups. They concluded that cross-reactions would occur after ingesting foods belonging to the same food family, similar to the cross-reactions observed in pollen allergies.

Recent studies by S. Allan Bock, M.D., and others at National Jewish Medical and Research Center in Denver show that this type of cross-reactivity does not commonly occur. Sampson of the Jaffe Food Allergy Institute in New York studied sixty-nine patients with one or more positive skin tests to legumes and gave them oral double-blind placebo-controlled food challenges in the hospital with five legumes: peanut, soybean, pea, green bean, and lima bean. Only two patients had a positive food challenge to more than one legume. They concluded that clinically relevant cross-reactivity to legumes is very rare and that clinical sensitivity to one legume does not warrant dietary elimination of the entire legume food family unless sensitivity to each food is confirmed by blind oral challenges.

There is one special consideration regarding other legumes. A recent report by Denise Moneret-Vautrin, M.D., from France demonstrated cross-reactivity between peanut and another legume, the lupine. The lupine is consumed either in the form of seeds or as flour used to supplement wheat flour. In France, apparently up to 10 percent lupine flour can be added to wheat flour and is not subject to labeling. Lupine flour is used in baked goods, pasta, sauces, milk, and soy substitutes. There have been several reports of lupine allergy. This study examined twenty-four peanut-allergic individuals for lupine allergy and found positive skin prick tests in 44 percent. In six people challenged by a double-blind, placebo-controlled food challenge, or DBPCFC, five were positive to lupine. The blood from four individuals demonstrated RAST inhibition to lupine by peanut, demonstrating cross-reactivity. The authors warn that cross-reactivity to this legume hidden in wheat flour can be a serious problem for the peanut-allergic individual. Read labels of imported foods, especially baked goods, for lupine or lupine flour and avoid them.

You can be allergic to multiple foods, including foods in the same family, but this is usually a result of separate allergies, not a common cross-reacting allergy. In general, you need avoid only the specific food you are allergic to by history; it is not necessary to avoid the entire food family. The two main exceptions to this recommendation would be the tree nuts and the crustacean shellfish (e.g., shrimp, lobster, crab, and crayfish). There does seem to be cross-reactivity among members of these food groups.

The rate of cross-reactivity between a tree nut with other tree nuts is greater than 50 percent. A recent study showed that walnut, pecan, and hazelnut constitute a group of cross-reactive nuts and belong to the same botanical subfamily. Cashews, pistachios, almonds, and Brazil nuts are another closely related subclass of cross-reactive nuts and of these, cashew and pistachio strongly cross-react with each other. Peanuts cross react with tree nuts 35 percent of the time but with legumes less than 10 percent of the time. Soybeans react with other legumes less than 5 percent of the time. The rate of cross-reactivity of wheat with other grains is 25 percent. With animal proteins, beef and lamb cross-react 50 percent of the time, fish species cross-react with other fish species more than 50 percent of the time, and shellfish cross-react with other shellfish 50 to 75 percent of the time, particularly the crustacean shellfish.

If you are allergic to peanuts, you should also avoid tree nuts, but it is safe to eat legumes. If you are allergic to one tree nut, avoid all other tree nuts.

Are peanut-allergic individuals also allergic to tree nuts?
Investigators studying peanut-allergic individuals have found coexisting tree nut allergies in 34 to 50 percent of those people, depending on the study. Among patients with tree nut allergy, 22 percent reported having reactions to more than one tree nut. It is unknown whether the coexistence of peanut and tree nut allergies is due to cross-reacting proteins or whether this reflects a general increase in the tendency to react to highly allergenic proteins in an allergic individual. This may not necessarily be specific allergens, such as peanuts or tree nuts, but may apply to all allergenic foods. This is supported by Sampson's study that showed that of the peanut- and tree nut–allergic population, 57 percent are also allergic to egg, 37 percent are also allergic to milk, and 29 percent are also allergic to fish and shellfish. People who are allergic to one food seem to have the tendency to be allergic to others. On the other hand, there is some evidence of cross-reactivity between peanuts, walnuts, and pecans.

Should peanut-allergic individuals avoid tree nuts?
Clearly, there are many people with peanut allergy who can eat tree nuts with no problem and many people with tree-nut allergies who can eat peanuts. However, many allergists, myself included, recommend that young children allergic to peanuts avoid all tree nuts. The rationale for this recommendation is the difficulty identifying specific nuts, particularly in mixtures and processed foods, the significant potential for peanuts to contaminate other nuts, and the recognition that tree-nut allergy is also potentially severe and lifelong. There is also the potential problem of confusion in the child's caretaker not familiar with food allergy and not being able to distinguish among the different tree nuts and peanuts; it is simply easier to tell those people "Do not give my child any nuts!"

Should peanut- and nut-allergic individuals avoid seeds?
Sesame seed allergy is becoming common throughout the world and particularly in Middle Eastern countries such as Israel. Rates of

sesame seed allergy are more common than peanut allergy and are exceeded only by milk and egg allergy. This most likely reflects the dietary practices of Middle Eastern countries where sesame paste is an important food like peanut butter is in this country. The allergenic proteins in sesame seed share some similarities to ara h 1, the major peanut allergen. The risk of having sesame seed allergy in peanut- and nut-allergic patients hasn't been carefully studied but is thought to be low, about 5 to 10 percent. Because sesame seed allergy can be associated with anaphylaxis and sesame seed is a common food ingredient, I often include it when I test a patient for peanut and tree nut allergy, particularly if there is no history of previous tolerance to sesame. If the tests are positive, I recommend avoidance.

Does soy formula cause peanut allergy in infants?

A 2003 controversial British study by Lack and colleagues raised the question of whether infants who consumed soy formula had higher rates of peanut allergy.

However, this question was resolved in a 2005 Finnish double-blinded study of 170 infants ages two to eleven months with milk allergy. The infants received either a hypoallergenic infant formula or a soy protein-based formula for two years and were followed for four years. At the age of four, there was no difference in the number of peanut-allergic children between the two groups. There was also no difference in sensitization to peanut measured by RAST testing between the two groups. The authors conclude that soy formula does not lead to the development of peanut allergy.

Can peanut protein be found in breast milk?

Peter Vadas, M.D., and his colleagues studied this question in twenty-three lactating women by feeding them dry-roasted peanuts and then measuring peanut protein in their expressed breast milk. There was measurable peanut protein in eleven of the women, with average peak levels occurring 1 hour after eating the peanuts. The peanut protein level had declined to negligible levels for nine women by 4 hours after, but two women had detectable levels at 4 hours and one woman had it for eight hours after eating peanuts. The amounts measured were very low but potentially high enough to cause a reaction in a peanut-allergic infant, and enough to cause sensitization in an allergy prone infant. I recommend that a nursing mother with a peanut-allergic infant restrict peanuts and peanut products from her diet.

Can peanut allergy be transferred from person to person?
In 1997, a case report was published in the *New England Journal of Medicine* of a liver and kidney transplant recipient who developed a new peanut allergy. His donor organs apparently came from a man who had died from peanut anaphylaxis after eating satay sauce containing peanuts. The recipient had no prior history of peanut or food allergy. Three months after his transplant, the patient developed a skin rash and swelling of his throat after eating peanuts. A RAST test to peanuts was positive.

Interestingly, a woman received the pancreas and other kidney from the same peanut-allergic organ donor. She never developed peanut allergy, and she had a negative RAST to peanut. She was challenged with peanut and had no reaction. The transfer of peanut allergy to the recipient most likely was the result of the transfer of white blood cells contained in the donor liver called B cells, which produce peanut-specific IgE. Similar transfer of peanut allergy with bone marrow transplantation has been reported.

Because transplant recipients take drugs to suppress their normal immune response to allow survival of the donated organ, cells of the donor immune system are not destroyed by the recipient. This allows cells of the immune system, such as B cells secreting peanut-specific IgE contained in the bone marrow, to survive, and these transplanted cells will perpetuate the peanut allergy in the transplant recipient. In contrast, B cells and other cells of the immune system capable of causing allergies are not found in the pancreas or kidney, so these organ transplants do not transfer allergies from donor to recipient. Blood transfusions present no risk of transferring allergies because transfusion recipients are not immunosuppressed and any donor B cells would be destroyed by the recipient's immune system. For organ recipients, the allergic B cells might eventually be destroyed as the patient's immunosuppressive drugs are tapered. For bone marrow recipients, the allergic B cells are an intrinsic part of the bone marrow, so there would never be any improvement in the transferred allergy.

Organ transplant recipients should be warned of the possibility of their developing allergic reactions if their organ donor has a history of food allergy.

Can peanut allergy be cured by organ transplantation?

Interestingly, just as peanut allergy can be transferred from an organ donor to an organ recipient as described previously, there was a report in 2005 of a twelve year-old peanut-allergic boy who, after receiving a bone marrow transplant for his immunodeficiency, completely resolved his peanut allergy. The bone marrow donor presumably was not allergic to peanut. This boy had a lifelong history of eczema and allergies to peanut, pea, and lentil. At the time of his bone marrow transplant, he had outgrown his pea and lentil allergy but not his peanut allergy as his specific IgE to peanut was still high, 23.1 kU/L. He had a successful result from the bone marrow transplant with no more infections.

Seventeen months after the transplant, his specific IgE to peanut was undetectable. A skin prick test to peanut was negative. He underwent an oral peanut challenge and was able to tolerate 8 grams of peanut. Since then, he has been consuming all peanut products with no problems. By suppressing the boy's original immune system, his immune B cells causing peanut allergy were destroyed and then replaced by the immune cells of the non-peanut-allergic donor. The end result is that boy now has the immune system of the bone marrow donor with no peanut allergy.

The investigators of this report conclude that although their patient's peanut allergy was cured by bone marrow transplantation, such a drastic medical procedure is not a viable treatment for peanut allergy. This interesting report give, much insight into the importance of the bone marrow cells in the mechanism of peanut allergy.

Will I outgrow my peanut allergy?

Jason, age 5, had peanut allergy diagnosed at age 1 when he developed hives from just touching his face with peanut butter. He was never exposed to peanut again and was strictly kept away from all peanut and nut products without any accidents and did well. His family never needed to use their EpiPen. He did not have any other allergy-related problems. Jason was about to enter kindergarten, and his mother wanted to know whether he was still allergic to peanuts. Skin tests to peanut and tree nuts were negative. He was challenged with peanut butter in the clinic and had no reaction. He can now eat everything without restrictions.

Most studies seem to indicate that peanut allergy, unlike allergies to milk, soy, egg, and wheat, are stable through time and not outgrown. The first study to address the question of the natural history of food allergy was by Bock of the National Jewish Medical and Research Center in Denver in 1982. He studied eighty-seven children with proven food allergies; fifty-six of the children were older than three while thirty-one children were younger. Age three was chosen as a dividing point for the two study groups because all children older than three, in the experience of the National Jewish Medical and Research Center, had IgE-mediated allergic reactions. The study was conducted with telephone interviews and follow-up DBPCFC.

The elapsed time from initial testing to the follow-up interview ranged from several months to 7 years. In children older than three, 19 percent of previously positive food challenges had turned negative at the time of follow-up. The most common foods to become tolerated with age were milk, egg, and soy. Peanut and tree nut allergies did not improve significantly. In children younger than three, 44 percent of the positive food challenges turned negative. Milk, egg, and soy again were the foods that were tolerated with age.

Bock concluded that older children diagnosed with food allergy tended not to outgrow their food allergies in contrast to younger children, especially those with milk and egg allergies. In several other studies, older children and adults have been shown to outgrow or lose their food allergies if they completely eliminate the food allergen from their diet. The exceptions to this are the highly allergenic foods such as peanuts, tree nuts, fish, and shellfish.

To address the specific issue of whether peanut allergy is outgrown, Bock with Atkins published a follow-up study in 1989 on thirty-two peanut-allergic children aged two to fourteen years. These thirty-two patients all had impressive histories of peanut-allergic reactions, positive skin prick tests, and positive DBPCFC. Two to 13 years after their initial evaluation, the patients were contacted by telephone and gave updated information on the status of their peanut avoidance measures, their most recent peanut ingestion (both accidental and intentional), resultant symptoms and treatment required, and any subsequent allergy evaluation testing that had been done. All patients interviewed declined requests for repeat DBPCFC. Eight patients had successfully avoided any peanut ingestion. Seven patients had follow-up skin prick tests to peanut, and all remained positive from two to ten years after initial evaluation. Twenty-four patients had accidental ingestions; all ingestions resulted in symptoms ranging from skin reactions (hives, swelling, eczema) to abdominal pain to runny nose and itchy eyes to wheezing, coughing, and laryngeal edema. No patient had a drop in blood pressure or anaphylaxis. The conclusion of the study is that peanut allergy is long lasting and does not appear to improve with time.

In 1998, Hourihane and his British colleagues studied 120 children ages two to ten years. They all had a convincing history of peanut allergy and all underwent an open peanut challenge. Twenty-two children were identified who had outgrown peanut allergy, documented with negative challenges. Fifteen of these "resolvers" were matched by age with fifteen "persisters," and features of their history and symptoms were compared as well as skin test and serum IgE results. The age of the first reaction to peanut, serum IgE, severity of reactions, and the number of reactions were similar in both groups. There were no cases of anaphylaxis in this study. The time interval between the last reaction and challenge was longer, but not significantly so, in resolvers than persisters. The resolvers also had negative skin test results or smaller results than persisters. The resolvers tended to have fewer food allergies.

Hourihane concluded that some preschool children with mild to moderate allergic reactions to peanut have an 18 percent chance of resolving or outgrowing the allergy. Follow-up of fourteen resolvers showed no reactions to peanuts on further peanut exposure. This study is consistent with my own clinical experience and that of others, which has shown that young children ages two to three who become allergic to peanuts only, with mild, non-anaphylactic symptoms can outgrow their peanut allergy.

Subsequently, there have been four other studies from 2000 to 2004 all confirming that for a subset of patients ranging from 14 percent to 42 percent, peanut allergy can be outgrown. In my practice, approximately 20 percent of patients outgrow peanut allergy, comparable to the range found in the above studies.

The children who become successful resolvers all had meticulous peanut and peanut product avoidance with no accidental ingestions. Sampson has recommended that children who had an isolated peanut reaction in the first two years of life, and who have successfully avoided any further peanut reactions for three years or more, be retested by specific IgE testing and if the result is low, have skin prick testing done. Depending on the initial reaction history, a challenge can ultimately be performed to document the resolution or persistence of peanut allergy.

In contrast to the young children with peanut allergy, other studies, including Bock's, show that when peanut allergy develops in the older child or adult, it does not resolve with time.

In summary, approximately 20 percent of children outgrow or resolve their peanut allergy. These "resolvers" all have meticulous avoidance of peanut with nearly no accidental ingestions, smaller skin test results, and fewer food allergies in total. It is possible that the younger your child is when diagnosed with peanut allergy, the better his or her chances are of outgrowing it. I generally test young children with peanut allergy annually with specific IgE tests to look for a trend in the levels. If they show a consistent downward trend, that child could potentially outgrow peanut allergy.

When should children undergo a peanut challenge to see whether they've outgrown their allergy?

David Fleischer, M.D., and his colleagues at The Johns Hopkins University and the University of Arkansas examined this question by doing peanut challenges on eighty peanut-allergic children with peanut-specific IgE levels of 5 kU/L and lower, regardless of their history. Fifty-five percent of these patients passed the challenge. When the investigators analyzed the results further, they found that for patients with specific IgE levels of 2 kU/L or less, 63 percent passed, and if their specific IgE levels were less than 0.35 kU/L, 73 percent passed. Skin testing was not assessed in these patients during this study. Children with levels of 2 kU/L or less were significantly more likely to pass the peanut challenge than children with levels between 2 and 5 kU/L.

The authors of this study conclude that for children age four or older with peanut-specific IgE levels less than 2 kU/L, it is reasonable to offer a peanut challenge as the chances of passing are greater than 50 percent. For doctors in office-based practices, like myself, I recommend doing challenges only for patients who have a very high expectation of passing. In my office, I challenge children older than age three years who have peanut-specific IgE levels less than 0.35 kU/L and negative skin tests. Ninety-eight percent of these patients in my practice have successfully passed challenges. For patients for whom there is a significant chance of having a reaction, I recommend the challenge be performed in a hospital setting.

Can a food challenge be wrong?

There actually is a false negative rate of 1 to 3 percent for food challenges. So, after a patient passes the food challenge, a normal serving of the food should be eaten under supervision just to make sure there is absolutely no problem.

Is there a chance that after I outgrow my peanut allergy, the peanut allergy may come back?

In Fleischer's study, as well as several other reports, approximately 8 percent of patients who had passed peanut challenges subsequently developed allergic reactions when they ate peanuts. There was no helpful information in the patients' testing or past history that could predict who would have a relapse of peanut allergy.

All the patients who relapsed had avoided eating peanuts while the patients who ate peanuts were much less likely to relapse. It seems that after resolving peanut allergy, the continued exposure to peanut in the diet confers tolerance to it but this tolerance is not maintained in the absence of peanut consumption. Therefore, after you or your child has passed the peanut challenge, I would recommend that you include peanut and peanut products in your diet 2 to 3 times a week. Because we still do not fully understand all the risk factors for who will relapse, I recommend continuing to have an EpiPen for a year, and longer if peanut is not consumed regularly.

Can allergies to tree nuts be outgrown?

Fleischer and his Johns Hopkins colleagues studied 278 patients age three to twenty-one years old with allergies to tree nuts. Almost two-thirds of the reactions were moderate to severe, and reactions to cashew and walnut accounted for nearly two-thirds of the severe reactions. Oral challenges were offered to patients aged four years and older, who had specific levels of less than 10 kU/L and no reactions to tree nuts in the past year.

Of the 278 patients, 117 met the challenge criteria on the basis of clinical history and specific IgE levels. Of these 117 patients, 78 declined to be challenged. The patients who declined to be challenged had significantly higher specific IgE levels, were more allergic to other foods including peanut, and less likely to have outgrown other food allergies. Of the thirty-nine patients who underwent oral challenges to tree nuts, twenty-three patients (9 percent) passed. As with peanut allergy, the specific IgE levels were helpful in predicting who would pass the challenges: 58 percent with levels of 5 kU/L or less, 63 percent with levels of 2 kU/L or less, and 75 percent with levels less than 0.35 kU/L passed.

Another conclusion of the study was that outgrowing peanut allergy was associated with outgrowing tree nut allergy. Having allergies to more than one or two different tree nuts decreases the chances of outgrowing tree nut allergies. Even though only 9 percent of tree nut–allergic patients outgrow their allergies, I recommend repeating the specific IgE levels to tree nuts annually for children and would consider challenges if the child is age four or older and has specific IgE less than 2 kU/L. At this time the rate of recurrence of tree nut allergy after it has been outgrown is unknown.

CHAPTER 3

WHAT YOU NEED TO KNOW ABOUT ANAPHYLAXIS

What is anaphylaxis?

At the party, George made sure to ask whether the sugar cookie he ate contained nuts because he had a severe peanut and tree nut allergy. The hostess assured him they did not since she baked them herself. As soon as he took a bite of the cookie, George knew something was wrong. He felt his lips, tongue, and throat instantly swell, and his entire body became intensely itchy. Within a few minutes, he felt chest pain and tightness, and he could not breathe. His face and body were bright red and covered with hives. He had the feeling he was going to die. He was able to reach for his EpiPen and inject himself in the thigh before passing out. Luckily his wife had already called 911, and by the time the paramedics arrived 15 minutes later, George had regained consciousness and could breathe. He received another dose of epinephrine and was transported to the local hospital, where he received intravenous fluids, antihistamines, steroids, and aerosol asthma medications over the next 12 hours. He made a full recovery and was discharged the following morning, completely back to normal. Later, the hostess of the party admitted that she had forgotten she had made the sugar cookies in the same mixing bowl that she had previously used to make cookies that contained nuts.

Anaphylaxis is the systemic manifestation of allergy—when an allergic reaction affects the body as a whole and not just locally. In other words, some patients have hives just in the area of contact with the food allergen, such as the lips and mouth, while other patients erupt in hives over their entire body, regardless of the route of exposure. It is this latter systemic total body reaction that is termed anaphylaxis.

A 2006 symposium of experts convened and a consensus was reached on the clinical definition of anaphylaxis. They established three criteria, any one of which was enough to indicate the likelihood of anaphylaxis:

1. An acutely occurring (minutes to several hours) illness involving skin, mucous membranes, and at least one of the following: respiratory compromise, reduced blood pressure, OR
2. Two of more of the following that occur promptly after exposure to an allergen: skin/mucous membrane involvement, respiratory distress, reduced blood pressure, gastrointestinal symptoms, OR
3. Reduced blood pressure after exposure to the allergen.

So a person who is having a combination of symptoms such as hives and vomiting with cramping abdominal pain, is undergoing anaphylaxis because two organ systems (the skin and GI tract) are involved, even if the symptoms themselves are not severe. It is the involvement of two organ systems or more, indicating the reaction is systemic, that defines anaphylaxis.

The severity of anaphylaxis can be graded mild, moderate, or severe. The symptoms of mild anaphylaxis can include hives, a sensation of fullness of the mouth and throat, swelling of the eyelids and lips, and nasal congestion. Moderate anaphylaxis would be accompanied by the additional symptoms of generalized or rapidly worsening hives and itching, swelling, flushing, tightness of the throat and chest, wheezing, and vomiting.

The potential worse-case scenario is severe anaphylaxis, which is a life-threatening reaction. This can cause severe swelling of the tissues of the upper airway, resulting in obstruction of breathing through the throat, blocking airflow in and out of the lungs. When the lower airways of the lungs narrow, shortness of breath, wheezing, and asthma can occur, compromising oxygenation. When the cardiovascular system of the body undergoes anaphylaxis, massive tissue leakage from blood vessels results in decreased blood pressure and shock. Severe anaphylaxis is explosive in onset, usually occurring within minutes after exposure. Patients often have a sense of impending doom in the initial stages of severe anaphylaxis. Seizures can result from lack of oxygen. The combination of obstructed breathing and lack of oxygen with loss of heart function and blood pressure is often fatal.

Grades of Anaphylaxis and Treatment

Severity	Symptoms	Treatment
Mild	Skin involvement only	Antihistamines
Moderate	Generalized or rapidly progressive skin involvement, throat swelling, respiratory distress, gastrointestinal pain, and vomiting and diarrhea	Epinephrine, antihistamines, emergency medical attention
Severe	Cardiovascular shock, turning blue, loss of consciousness, death	Epinephrine, antihistamines, steroids, emergency medical attention, intensive care

The common causes of fatal anaphylaxis are bee stings, drug reactions, and food allergies. Annually, there are 300 deaths from penicillin allergy, 150 deaths from food allergy, 90 percent of which are from peanuts and nuts, and fifty deaths from insect-sting anaphylaxis. By comparison, the annual death rate from asthma attacks is approximately 5,000. Peanuts, tree nuts, and shellfish cause the majority of severe allergic reactions to foods.

There are other conditions that can mimic the symptoms of anaphylaxis. Chest tightness and difficulty breathing can be a symptom of asthma, heartburn, or anxiety. A heart attack is sometimes very similar to an anaphylactic reaction, so prompt medical attention by a physician is crucial so that proper and appropriate treatment can be given.

Is anaphylaxis always accompanied by skin symptoms?

In the major studies of anaphylaxis in the medical literature, 80 percent of patients had some type of skin or mucous membrane symptom, typically itchiness around the mouth and lips, hives, swelling of the mouth, tongue, and face, flushing, and generalized itching. An anaphylactic reaction usually begins with skin symptoms and then rapidly evolves into a systemic reaction with other organ systems. However, up to 20 percent of patients with food and insect sting anaphylaxis do not have any skin symptoms at all, so the absence of any skin involvement does not rule out an anaphylactic reaction. I have seen a number of insect sting anaphylactic reactions begin with decreased blood pressure and shock first, only to be followed by hives afterward.

What is biphasic anaphylaxis?

Michael was on summer vacation with his family and had just had some ice cream when he felt ill, vomiting and wheezing. His mother gave him his EpiPen right away and drove him to the nearest hospital emergency room, which fortunately was close by. By the time they reached the hospital, his symptoms had resolved. He was given prednisone and observed for 2 hours. They concluded the reaction was most likely due to the ice cream cross-contaminated with nuts and that the vomiting had expelled most of the allergen. Because he now appeared totally normal, he was discharged with a three-day prescription for prednisone and Benadryl. On their way home, Michael started to break out in hives and began wheezing again and complained he couldn't breathe. Unfortunately, they had used their only EpiPen and did not have a second one. He was treated with his albuterol inhaler and Benadryl and luckily there was an urgent care clinic right off the highway at the next exit. Upon his arrival, he was immediately treated with epinephrine and intravenous steroids. Because of the late-phase reaction, the decision was made to continue observing him overnight for any more allergic symptoms. He did well and went home the next morning.

———

Approximately 20 percent of people undergoing acute allergic reactions experience **biphasic anaphylaxis** in which the initial symptoms are followed by a delayed wave of symptoms 1 to 8 hours later. These symptoms are usually similar to the acute symptoms of hives, swelling, gastrointestinal distress, wheezing, and decreased blood pressure. The mechanism of biphasic anaphylaxis may be continued absorption of the allergen from the GI tract and/or the formation and release of additional chemical mediators triggering secondary responses. Having a biphasic reaction increases the severity of the reaction and the risk for a fatal outcome. Ninety percent of biphasic reactions occur within four hours but the time course can be extended to 8 to 72 hours after the initial reaction.

The biphasic reaction does not respond to antihistamines. Steroid medications are prescribed to prevent biphasic anaphylaxis but unfortunately, they may not be effective. Because the occurrence of biphasic anaphylaxis is unpredictable, and medications may not be able to prevent it, intensive medical treatment in a hospital may be necessary. I recommend that if you experience anaphylaxis, use your epinephrine and then seek immediate medical attention at the nearest medical facility by contacting 911 or your local emergency medical services.

Medical observation for biphasic anaphylaxis should be for at least a minimum of four to six hours. According to Hugh Sampson, M.D., most biphasic responses will occur within that critical time period. In a more recent review, Phil Lieberman, M.D., suggests an eight-hour observation period. Sometimes in a very busy emergency department, you may be discharged before the four to eight hours are up. I suggest that if you and your physician are unable to convince the emergency staff to have you stay longer, do not leave the facility. Simply take a seat in the waiting area for the rest of the four-to six-hour time period. That way, if a delayed reaction does occur, you will still be able to receive prompt medical attention.

Can severe anaphylaxis be predicted?

Richard had seen an allergist for asthma when he was a child. He had allergy testing then and recalled being told that he was allergic to cats, dogs, dust, and pollen. He never had any problems with food allergy. As an adult, though, he collapsed while eating at a Chinese restaurant. He was brought to the nearest hospital emergency room and found to be in shock. Tests showed no evidence of a heart attack. His skin showed no evidence of any insect sting, and his lungs were clear with no asthma; he was on no medications. He recovered fully and was discharged in 48 hours. He was referred for allergy testing to rule out food anaphylaxis. Skin tests were positive to peanuts, cashews, and almonds. His wife remembered that on that evening, they had ordered beef satay with peanut sauce and chicken with cashews.

There is unfortunately no available test to predict who is at risk for a life-threatening allergic reaction, short of doing an actual challenge test. The size of skin tests and the severity of positive sIgE tests do not correlate with the risk of anaphylaxis. Anyone who is allergic can potentially undergo an anaphylactic reaction. Peanut reactions are often severe, even on the first exposure. Forty percent of first reactions to peanuts involve wheezing and respiratory distress. Eighty percent of peanut-allergic patients have had reactions involving difficulty breathing. Because of this, I prescribe an EpiPen to all my patients with peanut and nut allergies, regardless of history.

What are the risk factors for fatal anaphylaxis?

There are five factors that increase the risk for a near-fatal or fatal anaphylactic reaction: (1) not receiving treatment with epinephrine or not receiving it in time, (2) a history of previous anaphylaxis, especially episodes accompanied by delayed or late-phase reactions (biphasic anaphylaxis), (3) having peanut and tree nut allergies, (4) a history of asthma, and (5) being an adolescent or young adult.

Being extra careful about following your restriction diet, especially when eating outside your home, and having your epinephrine autoinjector with you at all times are essential. Ninety percent of fatal reactions occur within the first hour after exposure. If epinephrine is administered within minutes of the exposure, the outcome is significantly better. If you have asthma, make sure it is under control and that you have your asthma rescue inhaler with you at all times. Several studies show that up to 30 to 35 percent of anaphylactic reactions may be severe enough to require at least a second dose. Therefore, you should keep at least two EpiPens on your person. In addition, having two doses ready will cover the possibility that the first dose may misfire or be defective. Because one epinephrine dose may last only 20 to 30 minutes at the most, in the case of a severe, prolonged reaction or in the event of a delayed reaction, be prepared to administer a second dose. Teens and young adults have a greater risk of anaphylaxis because of the behavioral characteristics of that age group, in which risk-taking behavior and independence from authority are more common. I make it a point to regularly educate and counsel my patients in that age group particularly before they head off to college.

All peanut-allergic individuals and their families should be prepared to treat anaphylaxis. Because there is no cure for peanut allergy, strict avoidance and preparedness are the keys to management.

What is the treatment for anaphylaxis?

Dennis knew as soon as he bit into the cookie that something was wrong. His lips and the inside of his mouth began to itch and burn. His tongue and throat felt swollen within a minute, despite his downing a glass of water. He knew this was serious, and he had to get to his car where he kept his EpiPen. Running out the door, he started to wheeze with each breath. He was fumbling for his keys when he felt he was going to pass out. The last thing he remembered was injecting himself in the thigh with his EpiPen as he fell to the pavement. Fortunately, his next door neighbor was outside and called 911. The EMTs gave Dennis a second dose of EpiPen, which revived him and restored normal breathing and blood pressure. Dennis was brought to the local hospital where he received intensive medical care and recovered. He went home after 24 hours.

———

Clearly, avoidance is the best treatment plan. Documenting the exact allergens responsible for the reactions, and gaining understanding and insight into where the allergens are located (and hidden!) is the key to any successful plan. This is the subject of another chapter, which will deal with this crucial matter in detail. Once the allergic exposure has occurred and symptoms follow, certain steps need to be followed to prevent severe, potentially fatal anaphylaxis.

The first step is to recognize the signs and symptoms of anaphylaxis and determine that anaphylaxis has occurred. Once you determine that the person is having anaphylaxis, epinephrine must be given immediately. If the reaction is severe, and there is no immediate improvement, then assess for the "ABCs" of CPR (cardiopulmonary resuscitation) taught in basic first aid classes: "Airway, Breathing, Circulation." (See box below.) If the person feels dizzy or faint, lying him or her down with the feet elevated will maintain blood pressure and blood flow to the heart and brain.

The ABCs of CPR

Step 1: Check for unresponsiveness. Call 911.

Step 2: Tilt head back and listen for breathing. If not breathing, pinch nose, cover mouth with yours and blow. Watch for the chest rising. Give two breaths, one second for each breath.

Step 3: If the person hasn't responded, start chest compressions, pushing down 1 ½ to 2 inches at the breast bone. Do 30 chest compressions followed by 2 breaths, repeating this cycle until help arrives.

Ideally, elevation of both legs will help maintain blood pressure and blood flow to the heart.

Epinephrine given by intramuscular injection is the only drug treatment for anaphylaxis. Epinephrine is given for any symptoms that extend beyond the skin, such as swelling, choking, obstruction of breathing through the throat or lungs, wheezing, dizziness, vomiting, diarrhea, abdominal pain, as well as rapidly progressive hives spreading in a generalized manner. Uterine cramping and a feeling of impending doom have also been observed as signs of anaphylaxis. Any of these symptoms can be a sign of a potentially life-threatening reaction.

Epinephrine is the same chemically as the hormone that our adrenal glands produce in response to stress. It increases heart rate and blood pressure and in general prepares the body for trouble. In the event of an acute asthma attack caused by a food-allergy reaction, administration of epinephrine will quickly reverse bronchospasm and stop wheezing. Epinephrine will also stop the leakage of fluid from blood vessels and restore normal blood pressure and heart function.

These actions occur in seconds and are lifesaving. Epinephrine has a short duration of action and will usually wear off in 20 minutes. Therefore, in a severe, prolonged episode of anaphylaxis, it might be necessary to repeat the epinephrine injection. If the symptoms have not responded to the first epinephrine injection and are getting worse, the second injection can be given after 5 minutes. The use of epinephrine should be followed by immediate transport to the nearest medical facility for continuation of definitive treatment, monitoring, and follow-up. Epinephrine acts to stimulate the cardiovascular system, causing the common side-effects of this drug, which are increased heart rate, increased blood pressure, and muscle tremors. In case of anaphylaxis, an immediate health threat, it is always better to use epinephrine early, and to deal with, any transient side-effects from the epinephrine later.

Anaphylaxis cannot be treated, prevented, or masked by the use of antihistamines. Anaphylaxis is an explosive, rapidly progressive reaction that takes place in a matter of seconds to minutes, typically within 1 hour of allergen exposure. Epinephrine works in seconds and is the only effective treatment for acute anaphylaxis. Antihistamines such as Benadryl don't take effect for at least 20 to 30 minutes or longer, which is too late. Steroid medications such as prednisone take at least several hours to work, and have not proven to be effective in preventing late-phase anaphylactic reactions (biphasic anaphylaxis) even though they are commonly used for that purpose and also when there is an asthmatic component to the reaction.

Once epinephrine has been administered, a 911 call needs to be made for transport to the nearest medical facility. This is necessary for a 4- to 8-hour observation period to monitor for any signs of biphasic anaphylaxis. Because late phase reactions can be more difficult to treat than immediate phase reactions and can sometimes fail to respond to treatment with epinephrine, you should only be observed in a hospital where you can be provided with specialized and intensive medical care in the event of these more severe and difficult reactions occur.

Do all ambulances carry epinephrine?

Not all ambulances carry nor do all emercency medical technicians (EMTs) epinephrine have the training to use epinephrine. The EMTs who are able to give epinephrine have the highest training level; they are classified as EMT paramedics. The EMTs who have only basic training may or may not be qualified and licensed to give it, depending on the state you live in. Some states allow EMTs with basic training to assist the patient with his or her own EpiPen. Contact your local ambulance and emergency services and find out who will respond to your emergency call and whether or not the responding EMTs will carry epinephrine and have the training to administer it.

Food Allergy Research & Education (FARE, formerly the Food Allergy & Anaphylaxis Network, or FAAN) has been instrumental over the past few years in raising public awareness of this problem, and its efforts have resulted in most states upgrading their EMT training to include epinephrine training and administration and having epinephrine available in all ambulances. As of 2012, five states (Arkansas, Montana, Nevada, South Dakota, and Vermont) did not have most of their EMTs equipped and trained with epinephrine. Hopefully, with your and FARE's efforts, these states will work on changing their regulations and policies. You can keep up to date with the latest policy and legislative developments on FARE's website, www.foodallergy.org.

When should antihistamines be used to treat anaphylaxis?

When only the skin is involved, a rapid-acting antihistamine is often all that is necessary. Antihistamines block the binding of histamine to tissue receptors, which is what causes the actual symptoms of allergy such as itching, redness, hives, and swelling. For the treatment of anaphylaxis, antihistamines should be given *after* the epinephrine has been administered. Antihistamines can be useful secondary medications in treating anaphylaxis, but epinephrine remains the only first line treatment. Examples of antihistamines available without prescription are diphenhydramine (Benadryl), loratidine (Claritin, Alavert), cetirizine (Zyrtec), fexofenadine (Allergra), and chlorpheniramine (Chlortrimeton). Benadryl is commonly used for food-allergic reactions because it is effective for skin reactions and works rapidly, usually within 1 hour. It is a very safe medication, suitable for use by young children and pregnant women. Its main side-effect is drowsiness. Another effective antihistamine for acute allergic reactions is hydroxyzine (Atarax), which is available by prescription. It also has drowsiness as its main side effect. It is a good idea to have the liquid formulations of either Benadry or Zyrtec on hand because these are more rapid-acting than tablets, which need to be digested before entering the bloodstream.

Antihistamines relieve the discomfort from skin symptoms, any rash such as hives or flare-ups of eczema, itching, as well as runny nose, sneezing, red watery eyes, and cough from postnasal drip. Long-acting, nonsedating antihistamines such as loratidine, cetirizine, and fexofenadine are useful for preventive therapy of these more chronic symptoms and are available without a prescription.

Should I use my asthma inhaler if I wheeze from an allergic reaction to food?

Christina, age 15, was an eighth grader with mild asthma and peanut allergy. She was kissing her boyfriend, who, unbeknownst to her, had eaten a peanut butter sandwich 9 hours earlier. After several minutes of kissing, she felt difficulty breathing and yelled "I need air!" She used her asthma inhaler without getting any relief and ran out the door to get some fresh air. She collapsed on the steps and went into a coma from which she never recovered. She died three days later. Christina had never told her boyfriend about her peanut allergy. Instead he thought she had suffered a severe asthma attack.

Wheezing, chest tightness, coughing, and shortness of breath all are symptoms of asthma, but when they occur as an allergic reaction to food, you are dealing with anaphylaxis and not asthma. Therefore, the treatment for these breathing problems is epinephrine, not albuterol. The mistake of using the albuterol inhaler first is a very common one because, for most asthmatic patients, the reaction may feel like a typical asthma attack. You have to be aware of what exactly has triggered your chest symptoms, such as environmental allergies, the common cold, or having eaten a food you're allergic to. This is a key distinction to make, especially if you have asthma and food allergies, which is a very common combination. Studies show that not only is having asthma a risk factor for fatal anaphylaxis, but having food allergy increases the risk of fatal asthma. These are good reasons to keep your asthma under control.

Once the symptoms of wheezing and anaphylaxis have been treated with epinephrine, asthma treatment can be administered for relief of obstructed breathing. When wheezing occurs as a result of bronchospasm and narrowing of the airways in the lungs, inhaled medications called bronchodilators can be used to reverse this narrowing and restore normal breathing. These inhaled medications are part of the standard therapy for asthmatic patients. However, if you have food allergies but not asthma, inhalers might not necessarily be prescribed, unless you have a history of wheezing. Asthma inhalers are inappropriate in the treatment of anaphylaxis and should not be used to treat anaphylaxis without also administering epinephrine.

Special Caution for People on Beta Blockers

Beta blockers are a class of drugs commonly used to treat hypertension, migraine headaches, and glaucoma. They are also used in the follow-up care of heart attack patients and after surgery. Unfortunately, they block the beneficial actions of epinephrine on heart and lung tissue thus rendering it ineffective in treating anaphylaxis. Therefore, if you are taking a beta blocker, such as Tenormin, Timolol, Timoptic, Toprol, or Lopressor, consult your physician for appropriate alternate medicines.

What is the Epipen?

Epinephrine is available by prescription as a preloaded autoinjector, as EpiPen. A similar autoinjector, Adrenaclick, and a generic autoinjector are now also available. There are differences in the instructions for using each device, so make sure the pharmacy dispenses the device that you have been using and are familar with, and if not, contact your physician. These are user-friendly, disposable devices designed so simply that the patient does not need to measure doses or see the needle of the injector. The device is activated by pressing it into the thigh muscle and held in place for ten seconds to allow the medicine to penetrate. Another autoinjector, TwinJect, had been available, but it was discontinued in 2012.

You should be prepared to treat an anaphylactic reaction with two doses of epinephrine because four studies of anaphylaxis have shown that between 16 to 36 percent of acute anaphylactic reactions may require a second dose. The requirement for the additional epinephrine dose was for the initial reaction, not for a biphasic reaction. In one study of sixty-four anaphylactic reactions, 3 percent of patients required a third dose. Also, being a mechanical device, if the first dose fails to activate or is improperly discharged, an available second dose would be important to have as a precaution. Recognizing the necessity of having two doses of epinephrine available, the manufacturers of EpiPen sell it as a two-pack containing two autoinjectors.

How to Use Your EpiPen

Remove the gray safety cap. Hold the EpiPen with the black tip against the fleshy outer portion of the thigh. Do not cover the end of the EpiPen with your thumb! Apply moderate pressure and hold for 10 seconds. Pushing the EpiPen against the thigh releases a spring-activated plunger, pushing the concealed needle into the muscle and discharging a dose of epinephrine. You can use the EpiPen directly through clothing. Upon removing the EpiPen after the injection, you will see a short needle protruding. The beneficial effects of the drug will be felt within seconds. The most common side-effects are a temporarily more rapid heartbeat and slight nervousness.

What is the correct dose of epinephrine to use?

The EpiPen contains 0.3 mg epinephrine, while the EpiPen Jr contains 0.15 mg epinephrine. The dosage of epinephrine to use is based on body weight. Doctors refer to a formula: 0.01 mg per kg body weight, which works out to 33 to 66 pounds for the EpiPen Jr and greater than 66 pounds for the EpiPen. Interestingly, this formula is not based on clinical studies but has been in the medical literature for many decades. As a result, there is variability in the doses prescribed for patients; the instructions for epinephrine prescribing gives the doctor flexibility in dosing based on the particular patient's medical history. For example, for a child with a history of anaphylaxis and asthma, I would prescribe the EpiPen at a weight of 50 to 55 pounds whereas for another child who has never had any reactions at all, I would prescribe the EpiPen at a weight of 66 pounds. On average, for children who weigh less than 50 pounds I prescribe EpiPen Jr and for children weighing more than 50 pounds and for adults, I prescribe EpiPen. For young children weighing less than 33 pounds, according to the formula of 0.01 mg per kg body weight, the EpiPen Jr would technically be an overdose. Because there is no epinephrine autoinjector containing less than 0.15 mg, one option is to have the epinephrine manually drawn up in a syringe. Unfortunately, this technique is very difficult to learn and in the actual event of anaphylaxis, studies show that mistakes in drawing up the correct dose and in the administration of the syringe are commonplace.

Most experts recommend prescribing the EpiPen Jr to children weighing less than 33 pounds despite the potential for a higher dose. The side-effects of too much epinephrine are typically a high heart rate, trembling, headache, and elevated blood pressure, somewhat like the effects of drinking too much coffee. Like caffeine effects, these symptoms wear off after 15 to 30 minutes, are not harmful in children, and are generally well tolerated. When dealing with life-threatening anaphylaxis, I prefer to err on the side of giving too much epinephrine rather than taking the chance on the dose being given incorrectly or not given at all.

The EpiPen delivers only a single dose, so multiple EpiPens have to be available if more than one dose is needed. Because epinephrine has a 15- to 20-minute duration of action, prolonged, severe episodes of anaphylaxis may require repeat doses. Epinephrine can be repeated in as soon as 5 minutes if the anaphylactic episode does not respond to the first dose. These devices are easy to use, and a school-age child can be taught how to use them with minimal effort. The EpiPen looks like large fountain pen and fits in a shirt pocket.

The epinephrine devices need to be with you or your child at all times, particularly when unanticipated allergen exposure is likely such as when eating outside your home or in school. Most elementary schools require the epinephrine to be kept in the nurse's office, so there must be a good plan for the student to have immediate access to the medicine when the nurse is unavailable. Some schools allow the epinephrine to be handed off from teacher to teacher as the students change classes. Most high schools allow for students to carry their epinephrine and self-administer medication with authorization from a physician.

In summary, if you were to ever experience anaphylaxis, the symptoms could be explosive and rapid, evolving in a matter of seconds to minutes. The only drug that will work quickly enough to reverse this and save your life is epinephrine by injection. It is the only drug that can simultaneously reverse airway narrowing, tissue swelling, and cardiovascular shock. Antihistamines work much more slowly and have no life-saving properties, but they do effectively reduce the discomfort of itching and hives. Antihistamines *never replace* the use of epinephrine in acute anaphylaxis. Steroids are prescribed to prevent the development of biphasic reactions, which can occur hours after the initial reaction, but because they are not always effective, it is best to be observed in a medical facility for at least 4 to 6 hours. In the treatment of anaphylaxis, it is better to err on the side of giving epinephrine than not giving it. All physicians are well qualified in the diagnosis and management of anaphylaxis, so if you ever have a severe reaction, use your epinephrine and then go to nearest emergency facility for treatment. *Early recognition and early treatment are the keys to the successful management of anaphylaxis.*

How often can the epinephrine dose be repeated?

Although a dose of epinephrine acts in seconds and lasts 15 to 20 minutes, for a very severe anaphylactic reaction, a conventional dose may be ineffective or only partially effective in reversing the symptoms. According to the most recently published guidelines for the treatment of anaphylaxis, epinephrine can be repeated every 5 to 15 minutes depending on how quickly the reaction is responding to treatment. Furthermore, the current treatment guidelines allow a doctor the flexibility to give epinephrine even more frequently based on his or her clinical assessment of the situation.

Obviously, an anaphylactic reaction that hasn't responded to one or two doses of epinephrine requires intensive medical care and treatment in a medical facility, and emergency medical services hopefully would have arrived by the time you have given the first dose. If you are in a remote area where you cannot be reached by emergency services within 15 or 20 minutes, you do need to be prepared with multiple EpiPens.

Would giving epinephrine unnecessarily cause harm?

The side-effects of epinephrine are rapid heart rate, trembling, headache, elevated blood pressure, turning pale, and nausea. These side-effects usually last for a relatively short time, 15 to 30 minutes, and have no lasting effect. They are similar to the effects of caffeine. In young, healthy individuals, these effects are generally well tolerated. So, if there is uncertainty as to whether or not to give the EpiPen it is better to err on the side of giving it because the risks of not treating anaphylaxis are far greater than the transient side-effects of the epinephrine. For the special case of patients with a history of heart disease, particularly older patients with coronary artery disease or a history of heart attacks, epinephrine can potentially narrow the coronary arteries and trigger a heart attack.

This conflict of medical problems does occur. I have some adult patients with a history of both heart disease and bee sting anaphylaxis. If they are stung, they need to use their epinephrine to prevent an anaphylactic reaction. I tell them if they don't use it, they could die from the bee sting. If using the epinephrine results in a heart problem, we can treat the heart attack. We can't treat them if they are dead from the bee sting! Again, this type of situation is uncommon particularly in the case of peanut allergy, which typically affects younger but otherwise heart-healthy people.

What is the best way to store an EpiPen?

The EpiPen should be stored at room temperature. It should not be stored in the car glove compartment, where it can get too hot in the summer and too cold and even freeze in the winter. If the EpiPen has been left out in extremes of temperature, examine the fluid in the window—if it is clear, it should be alright to use. As an additional precaution when traveling with the EpiPen, it can be kept in an insulated container such as a lunch bag, to maintain even storage temperatures.

Because the EpiPen needs to be available for quick access for an emergency it should never be locked up. This is particularly important in the school setting where medications are routinely kept locked in the nurse's office. Keeping the EpiPen in a secure but unlocked location can be specified in the child's individual health care plan.

Is an expired EpiPen effective in treating anaphylaxis?

Obviously, you always want to make sure your EpiPen is up to date and not expired. As soon as you purchase your new EpiPen, look at the expiration date on the device and make a note of that date on your calendar as a reminder. You can also subscribe to reminder services that can send you reminders by email or telephone messages.

However, if you are in a situation where you have symptoms of anaphylaxis and the only EpiPen available to you is past the expiration date, as long as the fluid is clear, you should still use it. Depending on how long past the expiration date it is, it may still have some activity left. Using an expired EpiPen is better than not using an EpiPen at all. Of course, call 911 for emergency medical services and if the expired dose did not help, you would hopefully have prompt administration of epinephrine from the 911 responders.

What is the newest form of the epinephrine autoinjector and how is it different from an EpiPen?

The newest epinephrine autoinjector is called Auvi-Q. It was approved by the Food and Drug Administration in 2012 and was made available in early 2013. It is a novel device. It is an autoinjector available in the 0.3 mg and 0.15 mg doses like EpiPen. Unlike the EpiPen, its action is by a propellant, not a mechanical spring. The needle retracts after the injection, so no open needle is exposed in a device that has been used. The press-and-hold action takes 5 seconds, not 10 seconds for the EpiPen.

The most novel aspect of Auvi-Q is its small, thin credit card size and its audiovisual cues (hence its name Auvi-Q). When activated, a prerecorded message prompts the user with each step in its use making the injection process much easier and hopefully less anxiety-provoking. The recorded message is powered by a lithium battery so the disposal of a used device needs to be appropriate for disposal of lithium batteries. The only potential issue with widespread acceptance of Auvi-Q may be its cost based on its acceptance by medical insurance and third-party payers, an issue with most new medications in the United States.

Can epinephrine be given in any other form besides injection?

Inhaled epinephrine is available as Asthmanefrin, an over-the-counter asthma inhaler. In studies using inhaled epinephrine for the treatment of anaphylaxis, doses of fifteen to thirty puffs are needed to reach the equivalent dose of 0.3 mg epinephrine by injection. Estelle Simons, M.D., and her colleagues studied whether children could use the epinephrine inhaler and found that only 20 percent of children were able to use the right number of puffs necessary to treat an anaphylactic reaction. Eighty percent complained of a bad taste and difficulty taking ten to twenty puffs at one time. The study concluded that inhaled epinephrine is an unreliable way to treat anaphylactic reactions in children.

Simons and her group published a study in 2006 using a new, rapidly disintegrating epinephrine tablet administered under the tongue for the treatment of anaphylaxis. The study was performed in rabbits and found that the tablets were easy to administer, and achieved the same blood levels of epinephrine as injected epinephrine. Preliminary human trials with sublingual epinephrine are underway. This form of epinephrine is potentially a viable alternative to injected epinephrine in its ease of use and more precise doses can also be given according to the patient's age and weight.

CHAPTER 4

WHAT TYPES OF ALLERGIC REACTIONS RESULT FROM PEANUT EXPOSURES?

What is the smallest amount of peanut that can cause an allergic reaction?

Daniel was only three months old when his parents realized that he was allergic to peanuts. He was still exclusively breast-fed and had never been exposed to peanuts before. His father had been cracking and eating shelled peanuts while watching television. When Daniel cried, he picked him up to hold him. Afterward, he was surprised to see a swollen, red, hive-like imprint of his hand on Daniel's back where he had held him.

In most peanut allergy studies, the lowest doses of peanut that provoked reactions were in the range of 50 to 100 mg administered in capsule form. To give you an idea of how small a weight this is, 1 ounce weighs approximately 30 grams and 1 mg is 1/1,000 of a gram. An average peanut weighs approximately 500 to 800 mg, or ½ to ¾ of a gram. This means that as little as ⅕ to ⅒ of a peanut can cause a reaction.

Jonathan Hourihane, Ph.D., addressed this issue of how small a dose of peanut people will react to, in a study published in 1997. He and his colleagues in England challenged fourteen peanut-allergic patients with doses of peanut ranging from 10 micrograms (ug) to

50 mg. Remember, 1 microgram is $\frac{1}{1,000}$th of a milligram, or $\frac{1}{1,000,000}$th of a gram! The peanut was administered in the form of peanut flour in gelatin capsules. Six of these patients had reacted to crude peanut oil, indicating a very high degree of sensitivity. Only nine reacted to 50 mg, the highest dose in the study. No patient reacted to 10 to 50 ug of peanut protein. The lowest dose causing any allergic symptoms was 100 ug, in two patients who had mild subjective oral symptoms. The lowest dose of peanut protein causing observable allergic symptoms was 2 mg, a quantity easily reached by inhaling peanut dust. Two mg is approximately $\frac{1}{250}$th of an average peanut.

Marjolein Wensing, M.D., and colleagues performed double-blinded placebo-controlled challenges on twenty-six peanut-allergic adults with increasing doses of peanut to establish a threshold dose of reactivity. Threshold doses for allergy symptoms ranged from 100 micrograms up to 1 gram of peanut protein. Fifty percent of the study subjects reacted to 3 mg of peanut protein, which is approximately equivalent to $\frac{1}{8}$th of a peanut. The lowest level of peanut protein at which no adverse effect was observed was 30 micrograms.

That microgram amounts of protein can induce allergic symptoms suggests that the potential for contamination is quite high and that quality controls in the food processing, packaging, and manu-facturing industry as well as restaurants and food preparation estab-lishments, need to be reexamined. Peanut-allergic consumers of these goods and services need to be always wary of and vigilant about the potential for hidden allergens occurring in these tiny amounts in processed foods and eating establishments. This may well apply to other highly allergenic food proteins as well such as tree nuts, fish, and shellfish.

What is "airborne" peanut allergy?

Elisa, age 7, had only mild asthma symptoms, usually sports-related. She was allergic to peanuts but knew to stay away from them. Riding home from school one afternoon, she was seated next to her best friend, who had unwrapped the peanut butter and jelly sandwich she hadn't had time to eat in school. Elisa didn't think anything of it but by the time she got home 15 minutes later, she was having an asthma attack and needed to use her inhaler.

Allergic reactions are caused by food proteins. Proteins can become airborne when the food is vaporized by heat or when the food is ground up or pulverized. At cooking temperatures, the proteins convert from solid to vapor. When this vapor is inhaled, it can cause allergic symptoms. Cooking fumes in particular have been cited as triggers of asthma attacks and runny nose symptoms. The cooking vapors of fish and shrimp have been cited as triggers of occupational asthma for workers in the seafood industry. The cooking vapors of eggs and steamed milk have also been reported to cause allergic reactions. Other airborne food particles from cooking causing reactions have included string beans, lentils, and meats.

In a similar setting, if peanuts, peanut butter, peanut oil, and peanut sauces are being cooked, the vapors emanating from the cooking can cause allergic reactions. Airborne peanut exposure can also occur when enough peanut particles are released from vacuum-packed peanut snacks in a pressurized airline cabin with a recycled air ventilation system. In this situation, there is the potential for allergic reactions from inhaling the peanut particles. Another example of airborne peanut exposure is at a baseball park where peanuts and peanut shells are everywhere on the ground being crushed underfoot into small particles that are easily taken up by wind currents and become airborne. A gust of wind can expose someone to this peanut dust and cause allergic reactions.

Now, what types of symptoms can you expect from this type of airborne exposure? Usually the symptoms consist of itchy eyes and runny nose, not unlike an airborne exposure to pollen, animals, or dust in someone with hay fever and environmental allergies. For anaphylaxis to occur, the peanut protein must be ingested, come in contact with the mucous membranes of the mouth, or somehow find its way into the bloodstream such as through a cut in the skin. An open jar of peanut butter at room temperature should have no significant vapor phase and therefore should not be a source of airborne peanut protein.

Does having severe peanut allergy mean I will react to peanut vapor?

Airborne peanut allergy describes the route of exposure to the peanut allergen, not the severity of your peanut allergy. All patients with peanut allergy, regardless of severity, can have reactions to peanut vapor. The severity of a person's allergy is determined by his or her history of previous allergic reactions. If the previous reactions were anaphylaxis, the person would be considered to have a more severe peanut allergy than someone who only has had mild skin symptoms such as itching and rash. Having had an airborne reaction does not necessarily constitute having a severe allergy; conversely, having a severe peanut allergy does not necessarily mean that you have had an airborne reaction.

Remember, most airborne exposures result in itchy eyes and runny nose; anaphylaxis is rare. The reactions peanut-allergic patients get can vary from exposure to exposure. The severity of reactions and the risk of anaphylaxis can't be predicted by skin testing or RAST tests. It is this uncertainty that makes peanut allergy such a concern for all of us and why such care in avoidance and prevention is so important.

Can the odor of peanuts cause an allergic reaction?

Another way of asking this question is, "Is smelling the odor of peanut butter equivalent to the different types of airborne exposures described in the previous section?" Medical literature contains reports of people experiencing allergic reactions merely from smelling the odor of foods they are allergic to. John Carlston, M.D., an allergist from Eastern Virginia Medical School, reported in 1988 on a 28-year-old woman who had had sneezing and itching reactions to the odor of peanut and peanut butter since childhood. The allergy worsened with age and reached a point where nasal symptoms occurred when peanuts were opened on another floor at the far end of the building from where she was located. Subsequently, she developed severe nasal symptoms and an asthma attack after peanuts were served on the flight she was on.

There are other, similar anecdotal reports. In 1996, R. S. Dawe, M.D., and J. Ferguson, M.D., reported on four patients from the United Kingdom with anaphylaxis to "airborne peanut vapor." It is important here to remember that allergic reactions to foods are triggered by food proteins only. The chemicals responsible for a substance's odor are called volatile organic compounds, chemicals that are not proteins and therefore incapable of causing allergic reactions. For peanuts, the volatile organic compounds causing its distinctive odor are called *pyrazines*.

As an example of how the odor of peanut butter is not allergenic, several years ago a popular children's book had a "scratch and sniff" feature. On one page was a jar of peanut butter and when the picture was scratched, you could smell the distinctive odor of peanut butter. Naturally, there was great concern that this book could be dangerous for peanut-allergic children to smell. The book was subsequently sent to the University of Nebraska for chemical analysis by Steven Taylor, Ph.D., and despite the odor of peanut butter, the book contained no peanut protein and posed no danger for peanut-allergic children.

The issue of whether peanut-allergic patients could react to the smell of peanut butter was examined in a well-designed study in 2003 by Steven J. Simonte, M.D., and his colleagues at Mount Sinai Medical Center. Thirty children with histories of severe peanut allergy, all with specific (sIgE) levels greater than 100 kU/L and histories of reactions to smells, were entered in a placebo-controlled, double-blinded experiment. The placebo used in this study was soy nut butter. Both the peanut butter and soy nut butter were disguised with mint and tuna to hide the real smell and covered with gauze to hide their appearance. A measured amount of either the peanut butter or soy nut butter was placed 12 inches from the subject's nose for 10 minutes. The subject was then observed for 1 hour in a normally ventilated room. There were no symptoms of any kind observed in any of the patients. This experiment conclusively demonstrates that the inhalation of peanut butter does not cause allergic reactions.

Another study by Tamara Perry, M.D., and colleagues from The Johns Hopkins Medical Center analyzed the air around peanut butter, peanuts, and peanuts being shelled, and found no detectable peanut protein in the air samples. Although the testing methods might have been unable to detect very small amounts of airborne peanut protein, those small amounts would be unlikely to cause significant reactions and anaphylaxis.

A similar, more extensive study by Rodney M. Johnson, M.D., and Charles Barnes, M.D., in 2013 examined the concentrations of whole peanut protein and the specific peanut allergens Ara h 1 and Ara h 2 in the air samples of a variety of environments containing peanuts or peanut butter. Their experiment simulated real-life scenarios from which they collected air samples: spreading peanut butter, removing shells from raw peanuts, removing shells from roasted peanuts, pouring a cup of peanut flour, examining the air above an open jar of peanut butter and open bottles of refined and unrefined peanut oil, opening a single-serving bag of peanuts, opening eighteen single-serving bag of peanuts (airplane scenario), and boiling raw shelled peanuts. There was no detectable Ara h 1 or Ara h 2 in any of these environments. They found only one out of three samples in the air of shelling roasted peanut contained whole peanut protein at a very low concentration, but no detectable ara h 1 nor ara h 2. These environmental studies provide additional reassuring evidence that in the typical "real life" scenarios of peanut and peanut exposure, the amount of peanut allergen exposure is minimal and unlikely to trigger severe or anaphylactic reactions.

How then do we explain the symptoms that patients experience when they smell peanuts and peanut butter? Hourihane believes that many reactions to the odor of peanut are "a psychological aversion and a method of self-defense against true allergic contact [rather] than allergic reactions actually mediated by small volatile proteins." He does, however, state that it is not proven that "extremely sensitive patients would not react to the smell of peanuts and this problem needs to be taken seriously, especially in enclosed spaces and those such as airplanes that recycle air supply.

The medical board of FARE does not believe that the odor of peanut products would cause true allergic reaction, although it could clearly cause a panic reaction.

The physical reactions that people have experienced from smelling peanut may be conditioned physiological responses similar to the conditioning of the salivating dog to the sound of a bell in Pavlov's famous experiment. Almost any physiologic response can be conditioned, from rapid heart rate, flushing, itching, hives, and high blood pressure to wheezing. The peanut-allergic child has been taught from a very early age to stay away from peanut butter because of its life-threatening potential. The smell of peanut butter is therefore strongly associated with allergy as well as with danger and fear.

The common symptoms of an allergic reaction can easily be conditioned over time. In addition, the symptoms of a panic or fear response can mimic the symptoms of a severe allergic reaction: increased heart rate, chest tightness, and difficulty breathing and talking. Unfortunately, the symptoms of a conditioned physiologic response and a panic attack may be very difficult to distinguish from a true allergic reaction. When in doubt, it is prudent to treat the reaction with appropriate allergy medications if the symptoms do not improve or subside with reasonable care and reassurance.

For patients and families who remain very concerned about inhalation exposures to peanut butter, I have conducted an "inhalation challenge" similar to the one that Simonte did, described previously. I place an open jar of peanut butter in the same room as the patient, hidden behind something or placed behind the patient so it is out of sight. As a control, I use an open jar of jam or mustard. I have yet to have a patient experience a reaction. Once they see that there is no reaction, they feel much more reassurance about being in the same room as peanut butter. You may consider asking your allergist to conduct this type of challenge if the inhalation issue continues to bother your child.

What are the risks associated with the different types of airborne exposures?

According to Robert Wood, M.D., director of the Pediatric Allergy Clinic at The Johns Hopkins University Hospital, there are four levels of risk involving exposure to food. The greatest risk occurs during exposure to foods being cooked. The closer you are to the cooking, the greater the risk. The second level of risk occurs with the manipulation or disturbance of food, such as when peanut shells are crushed or swept. The third level occurs with exposure to peanuts in a closed environment with recycled air such as on an airplane. Although reactions do occur in this setting and have been reported in the medical literature, they are still considered rare. The lowest level of risk occurs in the setting where food is being eaten but not cooked, such as in a dining hall or cafeteria, unless there is direct contact with the food.

You need to consider the exact conditions of your environment and level of exposure and contact to determine your level of risk. How these conditions are modified will usually result from a negotiated compromise balancing your needs and the similar needs of other allergic people with the needs of the general public. The social and legal ramifications of potential situations in which the public needs conflict with the needs of the allergic individual have not yet been fully played out. These issues will be addressed more fully in a later chapter.

Can skin contact cause anaphylaxis?

The elegant study performed by Simonte on the effect of inhalation of peanut butter also examined the effect of skin contact with peanut butter on peanut-allergic children by the double-blinded, placebo-controlled method. The same thirty children with severe peanut allergy were the subjects of the skin contact study. In this study, the placebo was soy nut butter that was mixed with a small amount of histamine to simulate the itchiness that would be associated with allergic skin contact from peanut butter. A measured amount of either peanut butter or the soy nut butter placebo was applied to the subject's back for one minute and then wiped off. The area of skin contact was then observed for one hour for any signs of allergic reaction. Three subjects (10 percent) had localized redness, five (17 percent) experienced localized itching without any visible redness or rash, and two subjects (7 percent) developed a single hive. None of these mild local reactions required any treatment. The authors concluded from these results that 90 percent of peanut-allergic individuals would not experience systemic or anaphylactic reactions to skin contact exposures to peanut butter, just mild local skin reactions.

Can kissing cause anaphylaxis?

Kissing involving the exchange of saliva constitutes a form of oral exposure to a food allergen that has been consumed by the kisser and certainly can cause allergic reactions, including anaphylaxis. Over the years, there have been reports in the medical literature of allergic reactions caused by foods ingested by the kisser, including apple, shellfish, and peanut.

Jennifer M. Maloney, M.D., and colleagues investigated peanut allergen persistence in saliva after consumption of peanut butter. They found that ara h 1 levels were undetectable in 87 percent of individuals 1 hour after ingestion of 2 tablespoons of peanut butter on bread, without any interventions such as teeth brushing. Consuming a peanut-free meal several hours after peanut butter resulted in undetectable ara h 1 level in all subjects. However, teeth brushing or mouth rinsing 5 minutes after ingesting peanut butter left low but detectable levels of ara h 1 in 40 percent of subjects. This indicates that instead of immediately brushing your teeth after eating peanut butter, a more effective way to eliminate peanut allergen from the mouth is to wait several hours and then eat a peanut-free meal. Peanut-allergic individuals need to be aware of this fact and counsel their partners before engaging in passionate kissing.

CHAPTER 5

FINDING THE HIDDEN PEANUT PRODUCTS

How can peanuts and peanut products be hidden in foods?

Katherine, age 18, was a nationally ranked squash player at Brown University. She was also very allergic to peanuts. After defeating the Wellesley College squash team, she and her teammates went out to a popular restaurant near the campus to celebrate. She ordered chili but did not inquire about nuts because she did not think chili would contain any nut or peanut products. After taking a few mouthfuls of the chili, she felt ill but was conscious and breathing. Her coach drove her to the home of a nearby local physician. He found her in shock. He injected her with epinephrine and called for an ambulance, which took her to the local hospital emergency department, arriving at 9:30 p.m. Efforts to resuscitate her failed, and she was pronounced dead at 10:55 p.m. The cause of the anaphylactic reaction was peanut butter used to thicken the chili.

Manufacturers are required to list ingredients on labels, especially highly allergenic foods such as peanut. Careful reading of labels is obviously helpful and important but sometimes not enough. In the United Kingdom and Europe, peanut can be referred to as "groundnut," and peanut oil can be referred to as "arachis oil."

The following terms on a package label may indicate the presence of peanut:

Arachide (French)	Mandelona nut
Arachis oil	Marzipan
Artificial nuts	Mixed nuts
Beer nuts	Monkey nuts
Cacahueta (Spanish)	Nougat
Cold-pressed, expelled, or	Nu-nuts
expressed peanut oil	Nutmeat
Goober peas (slang)	Peanut
Ground nuts	Peanut butter
Imitation nuts	Peanut flour

The presence of tree nuts may be indicated by the following terms:

Almonds	Marzipan/almond paste
Almond extract	Mashuga nuts (pecans)
Artificial nuts	Nougat
Brazil nuts	Nut butters (such as cashew
Caponata	butter)
Cashews	Nut meal
Chestnuts	Nut oil
Filbert/hazelnut	Nut paste (such as almond
Gianduja (a mixture of	paste)
chocolate cream and	Pecans
mixed nuts)	Pesto
Hickory nuts	Pine nuts (piñon, pignoli)
Imitation nuts	Pistachios
Indian nuts (pine nuts)	Walnuts
Macadamia nuts	

Source: Adapted from Muñoz-Furlong (ed.). "How to read a label." *Food Allergy Research and Education,* 2004. Used with permission.

What to Watch Out for

Peanut butter is a popular additive in cooking. Cooks favor its versatility, because it adds extra flavor and texture to many dishes. Peanut butter is often used as a shortening or oil in recipes for many gravies. It can give a smoother texture to sauces and gravies. It is used as a thickener for many recipes. Peanut butter has adhesive properties that allow it to be used to "glue down" the ends of egg rolls to keep them from coming apart.

Peanuts, peanut oil, and peanut butter are commonly used in many types of international cuisines, particularly Asian. Thai, Vietnamese, Chinese, Japanese, Indian, Indonesian, Mexican, and African cooking are a few examples in which peanut and peanut products play an important part. Peanut butter is often used as a flavor enhancer in many Chinese restaurants. Sauces and toppings can have finely crushed peanuts mixed in without any visible sign of them. Peanut sauce is often included as a hidden ingredient in chicken marinade. Peanut powder is a listed ingredient in some vegetable soup mixes. One brand of gourmet popcorn has peanut flavoring to enhance its special flavor. Peanut flour is used in certain brands of frozen dinners. "Slivered almonds" found on some baked goods may actually be made from raw peanuts because they are much cheaper. Peanuts can be reflavored and pressed into other shapes such as those of walnuts and almonds.

Crushed and finely ground peanut shells can be part of the stuffing material of bean bags, "draft blocker bags" that go under doors to prevent drafts, and similar items. Leakage or breakage of these items would lead to aerosol emission of highly allergenic peanut shell particles into the environment. One of my patients had a systemic reaction, with hives and runny nose, after exposure to a bird feeder. The ingredient label listed "peanut hearts." Some arts and crafts projects in schools use peanut butter as an ingredient so make your child's teacher aware that these items can be a hidden source of peanut exposure. Also, read the labels on store-bought arts and crafts projects carefully.

The Importance of Cross-Contamination

Cross-contamination of food-preparation equipment, utensils, and cookware is an important problem. Because of the demands of a busy restaurant kitchen, cookware and equipment are reused multiple times for many different entrees. Very small amounts of food that may not be obvious or visible to the cook, particularly oils and liquids, may be left behind to contaminate the next entree. Studies show that for most food allergies, as little as 50 to 100 mg of food protein can be enough to cause an allergic reaction. However, because the peanut allergen is so potent, even 100 µg of peanut protein (10 times less) can induce allergic symptoms in patients.

Commercial food-manufacturing equipment can be a source of contamination. The production of nut butters, such as peanut and cashew butters, are often run on shared equipment. The nut and plain versions of many products are often processed on shared equipment. Fortunately, the food industry is now, for the most part, attuned to the reality of food-allergic consumers. It is usually standard procedure for equipment to be thoroughly cleaned between the production of different products, and many companies keep equipment exposed to peanut products separate from other pieces of equipment. Every once in a while, you will hear of a company recall of a product contaminated by shared equipment in processing or packaging. Consumers should keep abreast of news reports and alerts from the food industry concerning product recalls and warnings. An excellent source of this information is the Food Allergy Research & Education (FARE), which publishes a newsletter and is also online (see Appendix A).

Processing Additives

The term "hydrolyzed vegetable protein" used to be commonly found on ingredient labels. Fortunately, manufacturers now are required to list the source of the vegetable protein so the up-to-date labeling should read "hydrolyzed soy protein" or "hydrolyzed corn protein," etc. A peanut-protein hydrolysate has been used as a foaming agent in soft drinks and a whipping agent in confections. Hydrolyzed peanut protein is not commonly used in the United States because it is more expensive to produce than corn, soy, or wheat derivatives. However, in other parts of the world, peanut processing is less expensive, so hydrolyzed peanut protein may be more common in food manufactured overseas. Another problem with foods manufactured abroad is that labeling requirements are often inconsistent and less rigorous than in the United States. It would be prudent to avoid hydrolyzed vegetable protein when traveling abroad or when buying international foods, which have become available in many supermarkets.

Use Caution with These Foods

Below is a list of some foods that peanut-allergic people should be cautious of. You need to find out as much as you can about the ingredient list of these foods because they might very well contain hidden peanut products. This is not an all-inclusive list and you need to always read the labels of *all* foods.

Baked goods	Ice cream
Baking mixes	Margarine
Battered foods	Marzipan
Biscuits	Pastry
Breakfast cereals	Nut butters
Candy	Satay dishes and sauces
Cereal-based products	Soups and soup mixes
Chili	Sweets
Chinese food	Thai food
Cookies	Vegetable fat and oil
Egg rolls	Vietnamese food

Ingredients such as "Oriental sauce," "emulsifier," and "flavoring" may also contain peanut products. The possibility of cross-reaction with the legume lupine found in flour was discussed earlier. In general, be careful of processed foods as they have a greater potential for containing undisclosed or hidden ingredients including peanut products. Always read labels! I generally recommend limiting your intake of processed foods and eating only those with which you are very familiar. Learning to cook your own recipes with fresh and all natural ingredients is not only allergy-safe but healthier as well.

Intimidating though the preceding information may be, once you know what to look for and become familiar with certain brand names and ingredient lists, grocery shopping should be easier and more routine. But, don't forget to read those labels because food manufacturing and production methods do change! If you frequent a certain market, befriend the manager and have him or her special order items for you. If you frequent certain restaurants, let the staff become familiar with you and your dietary needs. Reward these establishments with your business. Once you establish a plan and routine, eating in or out should remain a pleasurable and safe experience.

Why aren't labels foolproof?

Joshua was diagnosed with milk protein allergy at age three months. He had severe eczema, hives, vomiting, and diarrhea after consuming cow's milk formula and dairy products such as cheese, ice cream, and yogurt. His mother found that a number of food items she bought at the supermarket that were marked "dairy free" and "Pareve" (Kosher designation for milk free) caused allergic reactions. These included baked goods, bread, and nondairy ice cream.

Labels obviously have to be read and manufacturers are legally required to follow specific guidelines. The Two Percent Rule of *the*

Code of Federal Regulations requires manufacturers to list ingredients that constitute less than 2 percent of the total weight, but they do not have to be listed in the order by weight. Ingredients in flavors or spices are not required to be labeled nor are incidental additives if they are not functional and in insignificant amount (generally parts per million).

An ingredient can also be listed as a "natural flavoring" to indicate a small amount of a food protein added for flavoring, without identifying the actual protein. An example of this is casein (a milk protein) added to canned tuna. On some occasions, a manufacturer will change ingredients without changing the labeling.

Labels can also be very misleading. For example, "nondairy" contains milk protein, "egg substitutes" are low in cholesterol and mostly egg white, which is the allergenic portion of egg, and Lactaid or lactose-free milk lacks the sugar but has the same amount of milk protein. It is still most important to know all the possible "code words" listed previously for peanuts, nuts, and allergenic foods that can make reading labels confusing. When in doubt, consult your allergist, Food Allergy Research & Education (www.foodallergy.org), or call or email the manufacturer or go to its website.

Should I avoid foods with labels that state "may contain traces of peanut" or "manufactured in a facility that processes peanuts and nuts"?

Unfortunately, there are no regulations in the food industry for these advisory labels on food products. This type of labeling is voluntary and varies from company to company. In most cases, the consumer is being warned that because of the manufacturing or packaging procedures in the production of that food product, there is the possibility of cross-contact of the product with peanuts contained in another food product being produced in the same facility. The actual peanut protein content of products labeled with these advisory warnings was studied by Susan Hefle, Ph.D., and her colleagues in 2007. Their analysis showed that 7 percent of foods carrying these advisory warning labels contained enough peanut protein to elicit allergic reactions. My advice is to avoid buying and eating that product.

What is the Food Allergen Labeling and Consumer Protection Act?

On January 1, 2006, the Food Allergen Labeling and Consumer Protection Act (FALCPA) took effect. This federal law requires the food manufacturer to disclose on ingredient labels the presence of the eight major food allergens in the product. These eight foods are milk, egg, wheat, soy, peanuts, tree nuts, fish, and shellfish. Any food ingredient that contains protein derived from the major food allergens, including additives and flavorings, are subject to this law. Exceptions are highly refined oils containing little or no protein.

The presence of the food protein can be listed as "contains" followed immediately by the food group, e.g., "contains peanut," or the labeling may list the ingredient immediately followed by the food source in parentheses, e.g., "natural flavors (peanut, almond)." The common food allergens will be identified on the label in plain English that is easy enough for a second-grader to read. The intent of this law is to eliminate the confusion caused by the numerous terms used in the food industry for the many different food proteins, often obscure scientific terms familiar only to food scientists (e.g., ovalbumin is an egg protein). The hidden food allergens in natural flavors, spice blends, dyes, and colorings labels will be clarified or eliminated. Although sesame is emerging as an important allergen, it is not included as one of the major allergens and is not part of FALCPA. Unfortunately, advisory or disclaimer type labeling such as "manufactured in a facility . . ." and "may contain . . ." will not be changed by this law and food allergic patients will still need to avoid food products with this type of ambiguous labeling.

Is peanut oil safe for peanut-allergic individuals?

Jane's favorite restaurants were Chinese, Thai, and Vietnamese, so when she was diagnosed with peanut allergy, she was crestfallen because she knew peanuts were a staple of Asian cooking. However, she discussed her problem with the managers of her favorite Asian restaurants, and they assured her that no peanuts would be used in cooking her meals. Unfortunately, she subsequently experienced anaphylaxis while eating a seafood dish at the Vietnamese restaurant. The entree contained no peanuts or nuts of any kind, but one of the ingredients had been panfried in peanut oil before being added to the main dish.

Whether peanut oil is safe depends on how it is extracted. Peanut oil is extracted from peanuts by one of two methods. The chemical extraction method extracts the oil by using chemicals, such as hexane, and high-temperature distillation at temperatures of 300°F or higher. The expeller extraction method makes use of purely mechanical means with an expeller device at temperatures from 150° to 200°F. This method has been referred to as "cold-pressed" because of the lower temperatures used, as compared to the chemical extraction method. Gourmet cooking oils often are extracted by this method because the oil is more flavorful and is considered more desirable because no chemicals are used. Once the oil is extracted, it can be further refined and purified by several processes that remove free fatty acids, soaps, peroxides, and other impurities that might affect flavor, appearance, or shelf life of the oil.

Several recent studies have analyzed the protein content of peanut oil extracted and purified through these methods. All studies show that chemically extracted and refined oils have negligible protein content and are not associated with reactions when consumed by peanut-allergic individuals. In contrast, the cold-pressed or expeller extracted oils contain peanut protein and can lead to allergic reactions. In general, the oils containing the highest protein concentrations and, hence, the highest allergen levels, are the oils with the lowest levels of refinement.

Hourihane studied sixty peanut-allergic patients, challenging them with crude peanut oil and refined peanut oil. None of the sixty patients reacted to the refined peanut oil, whereas six (10 percent) reacted to the crude oil. Another study showed that one brand of crude peanut oil contained 3.3 µg of allergenic protein per milliliter of oil.

Another problem with cooking oils, particularly in a busy restaurant kitchen, is the risk of cross-contamination of frying different foods in a shared deep-fat fryer. In addition, it is common practice for the same frying pan to be used for multiple entrées with the pan being wiped off between entrées.

Because of the significant variability of factory procedures, labeling ambiguities and inconsistencies, you cannot assume that peanut oil is safe.

As mentioned earlier, in manufacturing, peanuts and tree nuts are often processed on the same production lines resulting in cross-contamination of the final product. Because of these many possible problems, and the severity of the risk involved, I advise peanut- and tree nut–allergic patients to avoid all nut oils.

CHAPTER 6

KEEPING SAFE IN A PEANUT-FILLED WORLD

Should peanut snacks be banned from airlines?

Elaine is a 34-year-old woman who has had a lifelong history of peanut allergy. She has had anaphylaxis when eating in restaurants on four occasions, despite always asking about the presence of peanuts in each entrée, and has used her EpiPen each time, effectively treating each episode. On a recent flight to Florida, she experienced sneezing, runny nose, and chest tightness when peanuts were served to the passengers in her row. She took Benadryl, which was sufficient to relieve her reaction, and did not need her EpiPen. She was moved to another part of the airplane and arrived safely at her destination with no further peanut exposures and no further reactions.

Peanuts have been served on airline flights since the 1950s. As the number of peanut-allergic passengers increased and reports of allergic reactions to peanuts on airlines occurred, complaints to the U.S. Department of Transportation prompted an inquiry into this matter. In 1996, an abstract from the Mayo Clinic was published that found peanut allergens could be washed from airplane ventilation filters after 5,000 hours of flight time. Consideration of this study, as well as the Air Carriers Access Act of 1986, which guaranteed access to airlines for the disabled, prompted the department to issue a recommendation, in August 1998, that all airlines provide on request a three-row peanut-free buffer zone for a passenger with a medically documented peanut allergy. This resulted in a huge outcry from peanut farmers and politicians from peanut-growing states as well as many members of the public offended by a small vocal minority dictating policy. A number of airlines subsequently announced peanut-free flights on request for peanut-allergic passengers.

The table on the apposite page gives you an idea of the diverse polices of some airlines regarding peanut-allergic passengers in 2012. The information in this table was compiled with the help of Terry Furlong and Christopher Weiss of Food Allergy Research & Education (FARE). Policies are constantly subject to change, particularly with changes in the airline industry, so it is always wise to contact your airline well in advance before making reservations.

The debate that followed resulted in a reversal of this directive. The main objections were that (1) it was an excessive regulation on airlines and ignored the rights of the vast majority of air travelers, who are not peanut-allergic; (2) the directive unfairly singled out one allergen, while ignoring other potentially important allergens; (3) establishing peanut-free zones would set a precedent for all forms of public transportation. Legislation was subsequently passed that prohibited funding for the U.S. Department of Transportation to implement its peanut-free zone directive but encouraged a scientific study of this problem. The lack of scientific studies demonstrating that airborne peanut allergen caused peanut-allergic airline passengers to have allergic reactions was cited as one of the main reasons for not mandating such strict recommendations.

Researchers at the Jaffe Food Allergy Institute in New York surveyed passenger reports of allergic reactions to peanuts on airlines and published their results in 1999. Sixty-two of 3,704

Airline	Regularly serve peanuts?	Non-peanut snack or peanut buffer zone available upon advance request?
Aer Lingus	No	
Air Canada	No	
Air Tran	No	
Alaska/Horizon	Yes	Yes
Alitalia	No	
American	No	
British Airways	No	Yes
Delta	Yes	Yes
Frontier	No	
Japan Airlines	Yes	Yes
Jet Blue	No	
Southwest	Yes	Yes
Spirit	No	
U.S. Airways	Yes	No
United	No	
Virgin Atlantic	Yes	Yes

Adapted with permission from FARE, www.foodallergy.org.

(1.65 percent) participants in the National Registry of Peanut and Tree Nut Allergy indicated that they or their children experienced an allergic reaction to peanut while on a commercial airline flight. Forty-two respondents, with an average age of two years (age range of six months to fifty years), had an allergic reaction that began on an airplane. Thirty-five of the forty-two reacted to peanuts and seven to tree nuts, although three of these could have reacted to something that also contained peanuts. Twenty individuals reacted after ingestion, eight following skin contact, and fourteen after inhalation.

The reactions usually occurred within 10 minutes, and the severity of the reaction was worse for ingestion followed by inhalation while the least severe reaction was by skin contact. During inhalation reactions, more than twenty-five other passengers were estimated to be eating peanuts at the time of reaction. Inhalation reactions usually consisted of upper airway symptoms, skin rash, or wheezing. The researchers felt that eleven of the fourteen inhalation reactions were very convincing for true allergic reactions, considering the timing and pattern of the reaction as well as the symptoms experienced by the respondents. None of these inhalation reactions were life threatening.

The people notified the flight crews only 33 percent of the time. Nineteen subjects received in-flight medical treatment, including epinephrine given to five, and an additional fourteen received treatment on arrival at the gate, including epinephrine given to one and intravenous medication to two.

Airlines have had epinephrine as part of their in-flight medical kits, as required by the Federal Aviation Agency, since 1986. It has been suggested to the airline industry that flight attendants be trained in the recognition of anaphylaxis and the use of epinephrine. Flight attendants should also be notified of passengers with life-threatening food allergies. Passengers should be warned that the airlines make no exceptional cleaning methods for flights. However, the airline might make allowances for allergic people to preboard so they can wipe down their immediate seating area. Passengers should be given the option of allergen-free meals or, ideally, peanut-free flights, if requested in advance. Passengers might be permitted, and encouraged, to bring their own meals if they so choose. This would safeguard them from the possibility of cross-contamination with other meals.

None of these suggestions are policy yet, but lobbying and a strong group effort by enough people could certainly result in changes.

Ultimately, even banning peanuts and peanut products from all airline flights would not guarantee safety for the peanut-allergic patient at risk for anaphylaxis. Passengers, particularly children, often bring their own snacks and candies with them, and exposure and contact could easily result. There is certainly no way for airlines to prevent this from happening. The false sense of security such flights might engender on the part of both the allergic passenger and the flight crew could end up causing more harm than good.

The patient has to take the ultimate responsibility for being vigilant and prepared. The strategy of education and prevention is key. Patients, families, and their physicians can help airlines and their staff understand about peanut allergy, how to recognize and deal with the problems of contact and contamination, as well as the handling of an emergency allergy situation. There is no substitute for prudent measures of prevention in dealing with this problem. Families need to always take the initiative and call ahead to inquire about the availability of peanut-free flights.

It is a good idea to book the first flight of the day in the early morning, to improve the chances of flying on a freshly cleaned and vacuumed airplane. Ask for permission to preboard or board early to clean and wipe down the seating area. You or your child need to bring your emergency medications such as an EpiPen, a bottle of liquid Benadryl, and any other medications needed (asthma medications, eczema creams, etc) in a carry-on bag for possible use during the flight. Remember, not only can checked luggage get lost, but it would be useless if an allergic reaction occurred during the flight. Bring your own peanut-free food and snacks, so that you or your child don't get hungry and start being tempted by the peanut snacks and other foods of unknown composition. To keep your child from being bored and wanting to explore and wander all over the plane, bring enough toys, games, and other diversions.

What are some of the problems facing peanut-allergic infants and toddlers?

Matthew is a two-year-old boy, who first developed peanut allergy at age one year. He was exclusively breast-fed until age twelve months and was not completely weaned until age eighteen months. He had developed eczema on his face, arms, and legs at two months. The eczema seemed to flare after his mother ate peanut butter and then nursed him. On his first contact with peanut butter, when he touched some on a cracker, he developed swelling of his face, followed by hives all over his body, and required Benadryl and epinephrine in his pediatrician's office. He has been kept on a strict peanut- and nut-free diet since then, and his mother eliminated peanut products from her diet. He had no problems until he was kissed by a relative who had just eaten a piece of candy containing peanut, and hives erupted where he was kissed.

Infants and toddlers are completely under the control of their parents and caretakers. They are a captive audience because they have no control over their environment. How often they get into trouble is directly related to how carefully they are watched and cared for. A strict peanut free diet and environment can be achieved for this age group more successfully than for any other age group.

The ideal situation would be a baby who is exclusively breast-fed by a mother who is herself adhering to a peanut-free diet in a household with no peanut products. Daycare would be avoided completely or at least delayed until age three. Unfortunately, this ideal situation is seldom achieved and is a bit unrealistic.

Siblings who are not old enough to understand that peanut butter can be dangerous should not be given peanut products except under supervision, so that accidental contacts with, and exposures of, the allergic child do not occur. The major mistakes occur when care of the child is given over to people who may not be as knowledgeable about peanut-free diets, or who do not care to be. This is where you need to educate others about the seriousness of the allergy and how often peanut products can be "hidden." Any caretaker responsible for the baby needs to be fully trained in handling an emergency situation and the use of epinephrine. In a daycare setting with multiple children, it is the responsibility of the daycare provider to maintain a safe environment for all her charges. How this is achieved certainly will vary from provider to provider.

With very young, active children, playing with and touching each other, it is quite difficult to monitor every child. Although skin contact typically results in minor skin reactions and not anaphylaxis, young children often put their fingers in their mouth, resulting in potentially more severe reactions with the oral exposure. The chances for accidental contact and exposure increase with the number of children present. In an ideal world, the easiest way to maintain control would be to have a completely peanut-free environment. Because this is often difficult to achieve, it is up to you, as parents, to be in frequent contact with the daycare providers, to give them information, hands-on support, and help.

When looking at various daycare centers, inquire whether they have had children with allergic conditions, such as peanut allergy, and how this was handled. The more experience the daycare provider has had, the more confident you can be about the safety of your child. FARE has a special educational package devoted to daycare centers and preschools. The Allergy and Asthma Foundation of America (AAFA) has a new program training childcare centers on dealing with food allergies, asthma, and other common allergy problems. Your local AAFA chapter will also direct you to the nearest support group and to educational lectures given by community physicians and local experts. These resources provide invaluable sources of information and forums for sharing experiences and giving mutual support.

How do I keep my peanut-allergic child safe at school?
Consider the following facts: Food allergies affect 8 percent of children under three and 6 to 8 percent of school-aged children. Eighty-five percent of children outgrow milk and egg allergies during school age but only 20 percent outgrow peanut allergy by age six. The prevalence of peanut allergies in children in the United States tripled from 1997 to 2010. Peanut-allergic patients have accidental exposures and reactions every 3 years. Seventy-five percent of allergic reactions to peanuts occur on the first known exposure. Twenty-five percent of epinephrine administrations in schools are for people who have never had food allergy or anaphylaxis. Fatal food anaphylaxis occurs in 150 people a year, 90 percent from peanut and nut allergies. Fatal anaphylaxis occurs most often outside the home, in schools and restaurants. Given these statistics, every school needs to be prepared to deal with food anaphylaxis, especially from peanut allergy.

In 2001, following the death of a peanut-allergic student in Massachusetts, the Massachusetts Department of Education convened a Food Anaphylaxis Task Force, which I was privileged to be a part of. We discussed the growing problem of life-threatening food allergies in schools and the importance of having all schools be aware of this problem and have ways to prevent and manage anaphylaxis. After meeting over the course of a year, the task force published in 2002 a 76-page set of guidelines for all schools on *Managing Life-Threatening Food Allergies in Schools*. It is a detailed document that includes an action plan and recommendations for the classroom, cafeteria, school sports, playgrounds, extracurricular activities, and school trips as well as the school bus. You can adapt sections from these guidelines for your child's action plan for school. You can view or download this document from the website of the Massachusetts Department of Education at www.doe.mass.edu/cnp. Many states and even schools from other countries have used these guidelines as a template for their own school policies.

The key points of the guidelines are to (1) identify the student with the food allergy to the school, (2) have a written emergency action plan (EAP) in place for managing an anaphylactic reaction, (3) and have a written individual health care plan (IHP) in place for the prevention and proactive management for the student in all the different school environments he or she may be in, from the classroom to the cafeteria to the bus to field trips.

The emergency action plan is formulated by your physician with your input, based on your child's history. It specifies which symptoms to look for and which treatments are to be given as well as contact information and directions for disposition following the reaction. The school nurse usually has the responsibility for implementing this plan in the event of an actual emergency. This is discussed in greater detail in the section on the school's responsibility to you. The general principles of the preventive IHP usually include the following:

1. Avoidance followed at home should be applied to all the school areas where the student may be. Nineteen percent of anaphylactic reactions in Massachusetts schoolchildren occurred outside the school building, on the playground, school bus, and on field trips.
2. For areas where food is consumed, school staff and students need to learn and adopt proper hand washing, no food sharing, and the routine cleaning of surfaces where food is prepared and consumed to avoid cross-contamination.
3. For the classroom, students and staff need to become familiar with the concept of "hidden" peanut ingredients not only in foods but also in nonfood items that may be used in classroom projects in arts and crafts, math, and science. Reading the ingredient labels of foods, as well as other items such as bird feeders, pet feed, etc, becomes an additional responsibility of the school staff.

4. There should ideally be a full-time nurse in any school where there are students with life-threatening allergies. If the school nurse is unable to be on-site, he or she should be able to train a designated staff member in the management of anaphylaxis and the use of epinephrine.

5. Every student with life-threatening allergies needs to have an epinephrine autoinjector in the school. The epinephrine autoinjector needs to be available for quick access within several minutes of a reaction, and kept in a secure but unlocked location.

6. Emergency communications between all the student's locations (classroom, cafeteria, gym, playground, etc) and the school nurse and/or principal's office should be available. Students, families, teachers, and school staff should all be educated on food allergies, anaphylaxis, and general avoidance principles. The Food Allergy & Anaphylaxis Network is an excellent resource for educational programs for schools and provides many age-specific materials, including videos for children and a very useful kit for school staff and personnel.

Why does every student with food allergies need an individual health care plan (IHP)?

The IHP provides a comprehensive plan for the daily management and prevention of your child's peanut allergy in the school setting. Formulation of the IHP is ideally a collaboration between you, your physician, the school nurse, your child's teachers, and all school staff who are involved with your child, including the principal, food services director, monitors for the cafeteria and playground, sports coaches, and the school bus driver.

Every aspect of your child's daily activities should be assessed for potential peanut allergen exposures and how to minimize those risks and maximize safety. Specific strategies are often dependent on age, maturity, your child's ability to follow instructions, and his or her social interaction skills. For example, for very young children, touching things and putting fingers and hands in their mouth is common, so keeping table surfaces clean and hand washing is important. For teenagers, risk-taking behaviors can be a problem. Modifications of the IHP as your child grows older are necessary to reflect these developmental changes and growth, so an annual review with your physician and school staff is important.

What is a 504 plan and when should a peanut-allergic student have one in addition to an IHP?

Children with peanut allergy and at risk for life-threatening anaphylaxis meet the definition of having a disability and are protected under federal law. The Rehabilitation Act of 1973, Section 504, prohibits schools from discriminating against children on the basis of their disability and guarantees their right to a free and appropriate education. Section 504 provides legal recourse for students and families when they and the school are unable to come to an agreement on appropriate accommodations based on the student's food allergy management plan. The family can then choose to file a 504 plan with the school district and undergo a formal process of negotiations with the school. In my experience, 504 plans have typically been unnecessary as, most often, common ground is reached.

Are there formal guidelines on food-allergy management for schools to follow?

Massachusetts was the first state to publish guidelines for schools to manage students with food allergies and anaphylaxis in 2002. Subsequently, twelve states have followed with their own similar guidelines: Arizona, Connecticut, Maryland, Mississippi, New Jersey, New York, Pennsylvania, Tennessee, Texas, Vermont, Washington, and West Virginia. You can check with your state's department of education or consult the website of FARE at www.foodallergy.com.

What is the Food Allergy and Anaphylaxis Management Act (FAAMA)?

FAAMA was signed into law on January 4, 2011. It calls for voluntary national guidelines for schools to follow in their management of children with food allergy and anaphylaxis, following the lead set by numerous state guidelines already in place. The bill specifically allows for the U.S. Department of Health and Human Services to develop and make available to all schools in the country a voluntary set of guidelines to reduce the risk of anaphylaxis for children with food allergies, and to provide incentive grants to help schools implement these policies.

What is the School Access to Emergency Epinephrine Act?

Studies of anaphylactic reactions occurring in schools consistently show that approximately 20 to 25 percent of cases occur in individuals (both students and school staff) who have had no previous history of any allergy or anaphylactic reactions. Most guidelines recommend that schools have in place unassigned epinephrine auto-injectors for use in these situations. Otherwise, these individuals very likely could go untreated and risk fatal anaphylaxis.

The following eleven states already have laws in place allowing for unassigned EpiPens in their schools: California, Georgia, Illinois, Kansas, Louisiana, Maryland, Missouri, Nebraska, Rhode Island, Utah, and Virginia. Virginia and Nebraska are the only states requiring unassigned epinephrine in schools. Recognizing this is a national problem, FARE has been instrumental in encouraging federal legislation that would allow states to adopt laws allowing schools to have unassigned epinephrine autoinjectors available. FARE's efforts culminated in the School Access to Emergency Epinephrine Act, which was introduced to both houses of Congress in late 2011. Its status is still pending, and I recommend you support this bill by writing your local congressmen.

Should peanuts be banned from schools?

Mark, age five, is severely allergic to peanuts and has already had three episodes of anaphylaxis, one requiring hospitalization. He has been kept out of preschool because the family could not find a school that satisfied their stringent requirements. They are now about to enroll Mark in kindergarten and are requesting a letter of medical necessity from me and their pediatrician to ask that his school prohibit peanuts and peanut products from Mark's classroom as well as the school cafeteria.

The social and legal aspects of this question are very similar to those related to airline peanut exposure. Many preschools and some schools have in fact banned peanuts from the classrooms and cafeterias. It is more difficult to manage very young children who typically are unable to follow commands, and engage in more touching and "fingers-in-the-mouth behaviors"—hence, daycare facilities and preschools are more likely to be peanut free than schools with older children. School policies on banning peanuts have therefore depended, in large part, on the age and number of students affected in the school and community, the efforts of the parents to be heard, and the willingness of the school system and community to make accommodations. Because there have not been any clinical studies that examine the frequency of allergic reactions and anaphylaxis in schools that ban peanuts and those that do not, there is no evidence base for policy makers, leaving the issue both unresolved and controversial.

There are valid arguments for both sides. Peanut allergy is a potentially life-threatening condition; it would make sense to eliminate any possibility of exposure in a setting with young children who cannot be expected to understand all the problems of management, let alone the implications of having a life-threatening reaction. On the other hand, without foolproof methods of guaranteeing peanut detection 100 percent of the time, there is no way to enforce a truly peanut-free school. It would be difficult to do detailed inspections of all food brought into school by other students, assuming everything had an ingredient label, and most families would not be expected to have adequate knowledge of peanut allergy to be able to make school lunches peanut-free nor could they be expected to have that motivation. Some argue also that a false sense of security results from a school that claims to be peanut free, resulting in decreased vigilance and monitoring over time.

Older children who never have to deal with real-life situations of hidden exposures and cross-contamination because they have been in peanut-free environments at home and school may be at a disadvantage when they go to college and eventually are on their own. There is also the consideration of the children with other life-threatening food allergies. Do we also ban milk, eggs, wheat, soy, tree nuts, seafood, etc from schools as well to accommodate these other students? These are by no means easy questions to answer and are the subject of many debates in local communities. Fortunately, most schools and families usually are able to agree on very practical school plans.

In most cases, compromise solutions are reached, such as having a peanut free table or peanut free zones in the cafeteria or a peanut free room. Some schools have a designated peanut table or area where all the peanut products are eaten, leaving the rest of the cafeteria peanut free. These zone approaches are generally quite satisfactory because the actual risk in a dining hall with good ventilation and no exposure to the cooking fumes is very low, particularly for anaphylaxis. Of course, every effort needs to be made to minimize any sense of isolation for your child; your child should be able to pick several friends with safe lunches to sit with at the peanut-free table. Students are given age-appropriate education on allergies and what the consequences of anaphylaxis are. The dangers of sharing foods and snacks must be discussed. This education often must begin with the school nurse explaining these issues to administrative staff. For preschools and lower grade classes with very young, difficult-to-monitor children and classes with multiple peanut-allergic students, a peanut-free classroom might end up being an easier approach for the teachers and staff.

The key to the success of any preventive plan is access to, and the availability of, epinephrine. This can never be overstated. Without easy access to epinephrine in areas where food and eating occur, potential disaster awaits. This can be a problem, particularly for children who, because of their age, do not have permission to carry their epinephrine with them and are therefore dependent on the school nurse for their epinephrine. Many schools have to share one nurse, so an individual school may have the nurse there only a few days of the week. In this not uncommon situation, the nurse has the ability and legal authority in many states to train a designee in the use and administration of the epinephrine. This designee can be a teacher, principal, secretary, or any individual in the school able and available to perform this crucial function in the nurse's absence. You need to know exactly what the school nurse's weekly schedule is and to whom the nurse has designated the responsibility for administering epinephrine on the days he or she is not present in the school. Obtain this plan in writing from the school nurse and principal.

How do I keep my peanut-allergic child safe on the school bus?

Another issue is the school bus and whether the bus driver will have the responsibility for keeping the epinephrine and administering it in an emergency situation. Most school systems hire school bus companies on contract and do not own the buses, so the school does not usually have total control over the bus driver's responsibilities. The bus drivers may choose not to take direct responsibility for the specific medical problems of the students riding the bus. This is a potentially serious gap in your child's preventive plan, especially because the school bus is relatively unsupervised with respect to sharing food, snacks, and packed lunches from home.

In Massachusetts, a new law was recently passed requiring that newly hired school bus drivers be trained in the administration of first aid and the use of epinephrine autoinjectors. The law does not require training of bus drivers already on staff. You might want to inquire about regulations in your state regarding school bus drivers and the availability and use of epinephrine on buses.

A policy of no eating on the bus can prevent most food-related problems. For children with food allergies, seating them near the bus driver would allow closer supervision by the driver during the bus ride. All school buses should have a protocol to follow in the event of an emergency of any kind. The driver should have an emergency communications device to contact 911 or emergency medical services. You should find out what emergency protocol the school bus has in place. Be sure to raise this issue with school officials because they do have responsibility for this part of the student's day.

What are the most effective cleaning techniques for removal of peanut allergen?

A recent study showed that ordinary cleaning techniques are completely effective in removing peanut allergen from hands and surfaces. Using a sensitive laboratory test for measuring the major peanut protein ara h 1, Tamara Perry, M.D., and her colleagues at The Johns Hopkins University were able to measure the effectiveness of a variety of cleaning techniques on the removal of peanut allergen from hands, tabletops, and other surfaces in school environments. After applying 1 teaspoon of peanut butter to the hands of volunteers, they washed their hands with plain water, antibacterial hand sanitizer, Tidy Tykes wipes, Wet Ones antibacterial wipes, liquid soap, and bar soap. Hand wipe samples taken before and after washing showed that all methods with the exception of plain water and hand sanitizer left no detectable peanut protein. This makes sense as the hand sanitizer is alcohol-based and may not be effective in removing an oil like peanut butter.

Also, 1 teaspoon of peanut butter was applied to tabletops and allowed to air dry. The tabletops were then cleaned with plain water, dishwashing liquid, Formula 409 cleanser, Lysol sanitizing wipes, and Target brand cleaner with bleach. All cleaners were effective in removing the peanut butter except the dishwashing liquid.

The investigators then paid surprise visits to six preschools and schools. Two of the schools had peanut-free tables or peanut-free food-preparation areas and one school was completely peanut free. None of the eating or food-preparation areas had detectable peanut protein, including nine samples from designated peanut free areas. None of the desks sampled had any detectable peanut protein. Only one of thirteen water fountains had detectable peanut protein at a very low level. The investigators concluded that under normal circumstances of hand washing and cleaning methods with common cleaning agents, school cafeteria tabletops and desktops are unlikely to be significant sources of exposure to peanut proteins. This study is of great reassurance and reinforces the importance of hand washing and cleaning surfaces of tables and desks in students' school management plans.

What is the responsibility of the school to your peanut-allergic child?

Nora, age five, is asthmatic and had anaphylaxis to peanut butter when she was eighteen months old. She has had hives from being kissed and from contact with playground equipment and toys. She is now enrolling in kindergarten and the parents are asking my help in filing a 504 individual health care plan and the school district's attorney has asked me whether the family's request for a

Food Allergy and the Law

There have been cases of daycare centers and preschools denying admission to food-allergic children or refusing to allow the administration of epinephrine. *Food Allergy News* has followed the issue of food allergies and the apparent violation of the Americans with Disabilities Act (ADA) in several articles (1997; 6(3):3, 1999; 8(6):7). There is ongoing litigation involving a number of these cases.

The ADA requires daycare centers to "reasonably modify their policies, practices, or procedures when the modifications are necessary to afford goods, services, facilities, privileges, advantages, or accommodations to individuals with disabilities, unless the public accommodation can demonstrate that making the modification would fundamentally alter the nature of the goods, services, facilities, privileges, advantages, or accommodations." The Supreme Court has ruled that the ADA does not cover individuals with disabilities that can be corrected or reversed with medical treatment. It felt the intent of the ADA was not to cover "common, correctable impairments and that the person must be limited presently, not potentially or hypothetically." Food-allergic individuals were not specifically dealt with in this ruling but clearly, food anaphylaxis is neither "common" nor "correctable."

In 2012, the Justice Department ruled that severe food allergies can be considered a disability based on 2009 amendments to the ADA that concerned "episodic impairments that substantially limit activity." Students with celiac disease (who need to be on a strict gluten-free diet) at a Massachusetts college had sued their school because they were required to purchase a meal plan that did not accommodate their dietary needs. The Justice Department ruled in favor of the students. So even though celiac disease is not a food allergy, the management of food avoidance is identical to that of food allergies and the Justice Department ruling can be applied to food-allergic students as well, especially if the risk of life-threatening anaphylaxis is present. How the food-allergic patient and the schools are affected will become clearer as legal precedents are set with the cases currently pending in the courts.

special aide to accompany her on the school bus and in the classroom is medically necessary.

———————

A federal law, Section 504 of the Rehabilitation Act of 1973, states that schools must provide medical attention to children who need it, and that budgetary cutbacks are not an acceptable excuse not to do so. The school has responsibility for the child's medical needs during the entire time the student is in attendance at school. State and federal law require that parents provide the school with written documentation of the child's allergies and the physician's signed treatment plan and procedure to follow in the event of a reaction. These plans provide for prevention and proactive management strategies (IHP) as well as the emergency protocol to follow in the event of an allergic reaction (EAP).

The school nurse, or the nurse's designee in his or her absence, will implement the medical plan. The plan should be very specific and list the signs and symptoms to look for during an allergic reaction. Based on recognition of these signs and symptoms, the nurse or designee will be able to give treatment and medication.

Medication policies vary from school to school. Some schools restrict all medications to the nurse's office. Obviously, this could be a potential problem if the nurse's office is situated a long distance from the eating areas. Death from anaphylaxis can potentially occur minutes after exposure. Ideally, the cafeteria monitors will be equipped with epinephrine if this is the case. Other schools have the students' medications in a fanny pack that is handed off from one teacher to the next as the student changes classes. Most schools allow students to carry their epinephrine and asthma inhalers after age ten to twelve, with the written permission of their physician.

It is important for families to provide a **written emergency action plan (EAP)** to the school and school nurse. You should develop this individualized plan with your physician. This can be a one-page sheet with the following information:

Student's name and **personal information** (age, class, address, and home and emergency phone numbers, parents' names and emergency phone numbers, and the closest relatives or designees from the family to act in the parents' absence)

Physician's name, and phone number

Medical information: specific diagnoses, specific allergies, and all medications

Signs and symptoms of an allergic reaction:

Skin: itching, flushing, hives, swelling

Mouth: itching and swelling of the lips, tongue, mouth

Throat: itching, swelling, tightness of throat, difficulty swallowing, difficulty speaking, hoarseness, cough

Chest: cough, chest pain or tightness, shortness of breath, wheezing

Heart: weak, thready pulse, dizziness, passing out

Abdomen: nausea, vomiting, diarrhea, abdominal pain and cramps

Action plan:

1. If peanut product is ingested and only mild skin symptoms are observed, give (antihistamine, dose). If hives are severe or rapidly progressive, give EpiPen/ EpiPen Jr. If systemic symptoms or anaphylaxis occurs, give EpiPen/EpiPen Jr.
2. Call emergency contacts (mother/father/designee).
3. Call physician.
4. Call ambulance if emergency contacts or physician not reachable.
5. This action plan can be modified for the individual student according to his or her specific history and needs. It needs to be revised as the medical history changes and should be updated at least at the beginning of each new academic year. A copy of this action plan

should be kept with the epinephrine. FARE's Emergency Health Care Plan is a convenient form reproduced on the following page that can be used as a template for your child's written action plan. You can also download it from FARE's website at www.foodallergy.org.

What can parents of peanut-allergic children do to help keep the school environment safe for their children?

Personalize Your Child's Items

Pasting the child's photograph on the action plan sheet as well as on the child's EpiPen prescription box for the school nurse makes for easy and quick identification in an emergency situation. Another good idea is to have the younger child eat on a placemat that has his or her name, photograph, and diagnosis of peanut allergy on it to further minimize the possibility of mistakes. Printing companies can make stickers on which you can print your child's name, picture, and diagnosis. These stickers can very useful in labeling medications, lunch and goodie bags, placemats, and other items.

Michael's mother became very involved with the school as a result of her son's peanut allergy. She started by talking to his class and answering questions about peanut allergy and how it affected Michael. She then talked to parents about peanut allergy at PTO meetings. She joined the local chapter of the Allergy and Asthma Foundation of America (AAFA) and attended its meetings. She subsequently organized lectures and speakers and arranged special programs for the students and parents of Michael's school.

Food Allergy Action Plan
Emergency Care Plan

Place Student's Picture Here

Name: _____ D.O.B.: ___/___/___

Allergy to: _____

Weight: _____ lbs.   **Asthma:** ☐ Yes (higher risk for a severe reaction) ☐ No

---

Extremely reactive to the following foods: _____
THEREFORE:
☐ If checked, give epinephrine immediately for ANY symptoms if the allergen was *likely* eaten.
☐ If checked, give epinephrine immediately if the allergen was *definitely* eaten, even if no symptoms are noted.

Any SEVERE SYMPTOMS after suspected or known ingestion:

One or more of the following:
LUNG:	Short of breath, wheeze, repetitive cough
HEART:	Pale, blue, faint, weak pulse, dizzy, confused
THROAT:	Tight, hoarse, trouble breathing/swallowing
MOUTH:	Obstructive swelling (tongue and/or lips)
SKIN:	Many hives over body

Or **combination** of symptoms from different body areas:
SKIN:	Hives, itchy rashes, swelling (e.g., eyes, lips)
GUT:	Vomiting, diarrhea, crampy pain

1. **INJECT EPINEPHRINE IMMEDIATELY**
2. Call 911
3. Begin monitoring (see box below)
4. Give additional medications:*
   Antihistamine
   -Inhaler (bronchodilator) if asthma

*Antihistamines & inhalers/bronchodilators are not to be depended upon to treat a severe reaction (anaphylaxis). USE EPINEPHRINE.

MILD SYMPTOMS ONLY:

MOUTH:	Itchy mouth
SKIN:	A few hives around mouth/face, mild itch
GUT:	Mild nausea/discomfort

1. **GIVE ANTIHISTAMINE**
2. Stay with student; alert healthcare professionals and parent
3. If symptoms progress (see above), USE EPINEPHRINE
4. Begin monitoring (see box below)

Medications/Doses
Epinephrine (brand and dose): _____
Antihistamine (brand and dose): _____
Other (e.g., inhaler-bronchodilator if asthmatic): _____

Monitoring
Stay with student; alert healthcare professionals and parent. Tell rescue squad epinephrine was given; request an ambulance with epinephrine. Note time when epinephrine was administered. A second dose of epinephrine can be given 5 minutes or more after the first if symptoms persist or recur. For a severe reaction, consider keeping student lying on back with legs raised. Treat student even if parents cannot be reached. See back/attached for auto-injection technique.

| Parent/Guardian Signature | Date | Physician/Healthcare Provider Signature | Date |

TURN FORM OVER   Form provided courtesy of Food Allergy Research & Education (FARE) (www.foodallergy.org) 5/2013

EpiPen® (epinephrine) Auto-Injector Directions

- First, remove the EpiPen® (epinephrine) Auto-Injector from the plastic carrying case
- Pull off the blue safety release cap

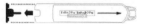

- Hold orange tip near outer thigh (always apply to thigh)

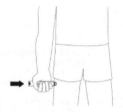

- Swing and firmly push orange tip against outer thigh. Hold on thigh for approximately 10 seconds.

Remove EpiPen® (epinephrine) Auto-Injector and massage the area for 10 more seconds.

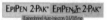

EpiPen®, EpiPen 2-Pak®, and EpiPen Jr 2-Pak® are registered trademarks of Mylan Inc. licensed exclusively to its wholly-owned subsidiary, Mylan Specialty L.P.

Auvi-Q™ (epinephrine injection, USP) Directions

Remove the outer case of Auvi-Q. This will automatically activate the voice instructions.

Pull off RED safety guard.

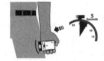

Place black end against outer thigh, then press firmly and hold for 5 seconds.

»)) Auvi-Q™
epinephrine injection, USP
0.15 mg/0.3 mg auto-injectors

© 2002-2013 sanofi-aventis U.S. LLC. All rights reserved.

Adrenaclick® 0.3 mg and Adrenaclick® 0.15 mg Directions

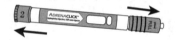

Remove GREY caps labeled "1" and "2."

Place RED rounded tip against outer thigh, press down hard until needle penetrates. Hold for 10 seconds, then remove.

A food allergy response kit should contain at least two doses of epinephrine, other medications as noted by the student's physician, and a copy of this Food Allergy Action Plan.

A kit must accompany the student if he/she is off school grounds (i.e., field trip).

Contacts
Call 911 • Rescue squad: (____) ____ -_____ Doctor: _____ Phone: (____) ____-_____
Parent/Guardian: _____ Phone: (____) ____-_____

Other Emergency Contacts
Name/Relationship: _____ Phone: (____) ____-_____
Name/Relationship: _____ Phone: (____) ____-_____

Form provided courtesy of the Food Allergy Research & Education (FARE) (www.foodallergy.org) 5/2013

Source: Food Allergy Resource & Education (2013). Reprinted with permission.

The most important part of any plan is communication and education, and here is where the family has a responsibility to the school. The major responsibility of the parents is formulating and submitting the IHP and EAP to the school. Ideally, the plan should be a collaboration among the child's physician, school nurse, and school staff. Entering kindergarten and first grade are big landmarks in your child's life. This is the ideal time to establish the educational messages that you as parents will ultimately be responsible for. Most problems that you and your child will encounter result from ignorance. Before school begins, meet with the principal and your child's teacher to discuss his or her specific needs as well as your suggestions for educating the class about peanut allergy. Find out if the school has had students with similar allergic conditions and whether or not they have had experience dealing with medical emergencies. You and your child can do an informal presentation to the class.

Contact the (FARE) about its school food allergy program; it provides an in-depth discussion for parents and school staff with a food awareness plan. There is also an excellent videotape available from FARE (see Appendix A) called "Alexander, the Elephant Who Couldn't Eat Peanuts" aimed at elementary school children. You can also offer to educate school staff, teachers, and other personnel with an in-service presentation. Invite the other parents, also. Consider inviting your pediatrician or allergist to be a part of this. I have gone to schools to speak with school nurses, teachers, and students about allergies. Often, the child's physician might be able to provide the in-service teaching as well. I have done this on a number of occasions and find it very useful for educating my patients, their families, and the school staff, and also for helping my management by improving communications, especially with the school nurse. The school nurse can be the "eyes and ears" for the physician and can be one of his or her most useful allies in caring for patients.

How will this allergy affect my child's emotional and social development?

Questions You Need to Ask the School

- Does the school have a full-time nurse? If not, what days is he or she there and who has the responsibility for administering medical care in his or her absence?
- Is the student allowed to carry epinephrine?
- What plan do you have in place in case of a medical, emergency?
- How many peanut- or food-allergic students have you had experience with? Are there any currently enrolled?
- Has the school ever dealt with an anaphylactic reaction? What was the outcome?
- What is the closest hospital that a sick student would be transported to?
- Is the cafeteria peanut free? Would you be willing to provide a peanut-free zone?
- If my child is the victim of a bully or harassment, how would you deal with that problem?
- Can we, as parents, set up an educational forum or discussion group to help educate students, teachers, and staff about peanut allergy?

Michael, aged seven has had a lifelong history of peanut allergy as well as allergies to tree nuts, dairy products, and eggs. At age five, he had a severe anaphylactic reaction at a birthday party, most likely to nuts. He eats school lunch in a special room separate from the main cafeteria that is "allergy free." He also has asthma, which requires him to use multiple medications during school hours. He dislikes gym and has refrained from participating in team sports.

He is constantly teased by classmates and is called "Peter Pan" and the "peanut man." Michael's parents are concerned that he is withdrawing and is depressed and they are consulting a psychologist to counsel him.

One of the more difficult challenges of having a child with a serious and potentially fatal medical problem is the general lack of knowledge that he or she will encounter in the other students and their families. Most people don't understand how dangerous food allergies can be. They also tend to be unaware of the concepts of hidden allergens, cross-contamination, and the fact that very small amounts of an allergenic food can do as much harm as the amount normally eaten at a meal.

People feel imposed upon when they have to make personal concessions to situations they do not fully comprehend. They may feel that you are overprotective when you ask that peanuts be removed from your child's environment. Therefore, education of the child's classmates and their families is just as important as the education of the school and its staff. This can be accomplished in many ways, both in the classroom and outside school. Meeting face to face with people is generally the most effective way of achieving cooperation. You can arrange to be on the agenda for the next PTO meeting, or invite parents to the classroom, or school cafeteria, where some of these potential problems can be made more obvious.

Besides lack of knowledge and ignorance, the other common problem many children face is that of teasing and harassment. Being "different" is likely to make youngsters the target of harassment by other children, and food allergy can easily make your child the prey of a bully. Recent studies show that nearly half of food-allergic children are bullied, the bullying is specifically because of the food allergy, and often bullying occurs with the foods used as threats. Quality of life was significantly decreased by bullying for both the child and parents. One study showed that parents were aware of the bullying in only half of the cases. This finding shows how important it is for parents to talk to their children often about their school experience and any problems they may be having.

Unfortunately, there have been many instances of peanut-allergic children not only being teased but also being physically threatened by other children. There was an example of a bully thrusting an open jar of peanut butter in the face of someone with peanut allergy. The life-threatening potential of this situation makes it more serious than just dealing with another bully, and the consequences are more much more severe than just hurt feelings. This behavior must be dealt with in a swift, definitive way, and with the direct involvement of the school principal.

With the recent attention bullying has received in the media, schools should be very responsive to any concerns, particularly with the life-threatening implications in peanut-allergic bullying victims. Under no circumstances should the child be given the responsibility of dealing with the bully or asked to simply ignore the bully. A face-to-face meeting with the offending child's family might be one way to stop this behavior. Many children are unable to comprehend death, and life-threatening scenarios may be too abstract for them to understand, so they don't realize the consequences of their actions and behavior.

Another consequence of having a serious and potentially fatal medical problem, such as peanut allergy, is in the fear and anxiety that it generates. Multiple studies show significant decreases in quality of life measured by standardized testing in patients and parents of children with food allergies.

Particularly in children, phobias toward eating can result, especially if the child has experienced a severe allergic reaction already. It is important that the child understand that while being careful is good, once safe foods are identified, they can be eaten without fear. Most fears in an older child can be overcome with patience, understanding, and reasoning. In young children, fear can be overcome with support and with the child knowing that there is always someone there to help if he or she gets sick. Your child's teacher, school nurse, and principal can be your surrogates during school hours; familiarizing these persons not only with your child's medical needs but also his or her specific fears will give your child confidence in them and ultimately enable him or her to develop self-confidence.

Because some schools have their food-allergic students sit at special allergy- or peanut-free tables, these children are separated from their friends and often feel isolated and even punished. Friendships and relationships often suffer as a result. However, many loyal friends will bring peanut-free lunches so they can sit at the table. Again, appropriate education of all involved is the most effective way to prevent problems.

Children often use their medical problems as an attention-getting device, and food allergies are no exception. They may claim that they are experiencing active symptoms such as "trouble breathing," "throat closing," "chest pain or tightness," "abdominal pain," and "uncontrollable itching," caused by their allergies. Address these symptoms early on and recognize whether or not they are truly allergic reactions. You have to be certain that there was actual peanut exposure associated with these symptoms. Physical signs of an allergic reaction, when present, are important in documenting a true allergic reaction. The presence of redness, rash, hives, and swelling can be helpful. You can substantiate symptoms that involve breathing difficulties and asthma with a measurement of lung function with a peak flow meter.

Bear in mind, however, that anaphylaxis need not always present with these symptoms, so the severity and urgency of each episode needs to be carefully evaluated by someone with expertise, such as the school nurse. If the attention-getting symptoms are rewarded with attention, your child may develop a behavior pattern that will make it very difficult to evaluate future reactions that are genuinely a result of peanut exposure. Professional counseling should be considered if your child's food allergy problem is complicated by this issue.

What are some of the problems unique to the peanut-allergic adolescent?

Jennifer, age 16, has had peanut allergy since age 4 and has not had any problems with restricting peanut and peanut products. She had a recent allergic reaction when her new boyfriend kissed her after eating peanut butter candy, and she developed facial hives. She is very upset today because her boyfriend doesn't seem to understand the seriousness of her allergy and has announced that he shouldn't have to "put up with this" and is breaking up with her. She "wishes she would die and be over with this."

In addition to all of the previously discussed issues, the adolescent presents a unique set of problems. We've already discussed the issue of kissing and peanut allergy in chapter 4. We're all too familiar with the mood swings and occasional rebellious "acting out" behavior of teenagers. A study by H. Monks and colleagues showed significant risk-taking behaviors by teenagers, including not carrying their EpiPens and eating foods with advisory warning labels ("may contain peanut . . ."). Some had inadequate knowledge of how to treat allergic reactions.

All adolescents seek some measure of control and a feeling that they can be independent. Many adolescents express this by deliberate actions to test the limits that have previously been set for them. For the food-allergic adolescent, this may sometimes take the form of either denial or rejection of their allergic condition and ignoring the restrictions placed on them. Such seemingly self-destructive behavior in adolescents is a common problem observed for the entire range of medical problems, from diabetes to asthma to smoking to drug and alcohol abuse.

Adolescents value belonging to their peer group and will try to avoid being cast as "different." They may feel embarrassed telling a

KEEPING SAFE IN A PEANUT-FILLED WORLD

new friend, particularly of the opposite sex, of medical problems such as a food allergy, which might limit where they could go out and have fun. For all the above reasons, the teenage years are actually when more anaphylaxis resulting from accidental exposures occur. A helpful approach might be to involve for support friends and peers who might share similar medical problems as well as the adolescent's personal physician or anyone else he or she trusts and respects. Giving the adolescents as much responsibility and control of their lives as possible will reinforce the feeling of trust and confidence they need, as they reach for adulthood.

For the at-risk adolescent who already has a tendency toward eating disorders, being on a restricted diet and avoiding food for medical reasons may worsen this problem. Again, early recognition of these issues and counseling will help prevent escalation of these problems. Self-destructive behavior or evidence of eating disorders clearly warrants consultation with a professional counselor.

I have found that a number of my patients who did well through high school had their first accidental exposures and anaphylaxis during their freshman year of college. This is usually the first time your child will be completely independent and has to make choices and decisions without you close by. In a new environment that includes new eating places with no food allergy restrictions, new friends, and new temptations, it can be difficult for the previously sheltered child to make the transition. Just as adolescence is the time to prepare socially, emotionally, physically, and intellectually for eventual adulthood, it is also the time for food-allergic adolescents to prepare to be on their own and to be able to deal with their allergies independently.

Certainly, high school is the time to begin this preparation by giving them gradual control. By the time your adolescent is ready to go off to live alone, he or she should be ready for independent living. When looking at colleges in the junior and senior years of high school, visit campuses and inquire about the food services as well as the health services and infirmary. Once the college has been selected, consult the local allergist so that he or she knows your child in the event of a problem. Meet the medical staff and show them your emergency action plan. Forward your child's medical records, especially those of your allergist.

Should you wear a Medic-Alert bracelet?

The Medic-Alert bracelet is a metal tag engraved with an individual's name and vital information in case of emergency, usually the diagnosis, allergies, and brief instructions. The tag can be worn as a bracelet around the wrist or on a chain around the neck. Its purpose is to provide life-saving information in case the patient is unable to give it because of either age or incapacity. In addition, the responding person can call the Medic Alert's 24-hour emergency response center, which has a computerized data file on the person with medical history and other vital information. Obviously, in the event of loss of consciousness due to anaphylaxis, a passerby can be immediately informed of the patient's diagnosis by reading the Medic-Alert bracelet and, if so instructed, administer life-saving epinephrine.

Whether or not a peanut-allergic patient chooses to wear the Medic-Alert bracelet depends on the risk of fatal anaphylaxis and the risk of the patient being incapacitated to the point where he or she is incapable of self-administering the epinephrine or communicating with other people. The use of the Medic-Alert bracelet in very young children would be for the remote possibility of their being left alone without adult supervision. A young child should always be under the supervision of a responsible adult who is well versed in the child's specific allergic condition and the management of an allergic reaction, including the use of epinephrine.

Of greater concern is the young child who is not quite old enough to understand and articulate the specific problem but is just old enough so that he or she might not always be under constant adult supervision. This is the child at the greatest risk for an accidental ingestion, often resulting from sharing and playing with other children. This age group is usually the late preschool to early elementary school grade level. Generally, older children and adults do not have any of these issues and the main reason for wearing the Medic-Alert bracelet would be in case of encountering the situation where loss of consciousness or incapacity occurs. The Medic-Alert bracelet comes in several sizes and styles and can be fairly unobtrusive. You can obtain ordering information from your doctor or contact Medic-Alert directly by calling 888.633.4298, writing to 2323 Colorado Avenue, Turlock, CA 95382, or at medicalert.org.

CHAPTER 7

PREVENTION OF PEANUT AND OTHER FOOD ALLERGIES

Should you avoid consuming peanuts and other allergenic foods during pregnancy?

Jill had a craving for peanut butter during her first pregnancy and admitted that every chance she had, she ate peanut butter sandwiches and peanut butter with crackers, cookies, and fruit. Her love for peanut butter continued through the three-month period she nursed her baby. Gregory, now two, developed peanut-allergy symptoms the very first time he was exposed, with hives on his mouth and face. Jill just found out that she is pregnant again, and wants to know whether she should eliminate peanut products from her diet.

Because allergic diseases, which include not only food allergy but allergic rhinitis (hay fever), asthma, and eczema, are all genetic and inherited, the baby who has relatives with these allergic diseases is at a greater risk for developing allergic diseases. If one of your parents has allergies, your chance of developing allergies is about 33 percent. If both of your parents have allergies, your chance of developing allergies is about 66 percent. A child's risk of being allergic to peanut if his or her sibling has peanut allergy is 7 percent. If the sibling is an identical twin, the risk is 66 percent. It has been a goal for pediatricians to prevent the development of allergies, such as food allergy, in infants with a genetic risk. This type of preventive strategy has focused on either the maternal diet during pregnancy or the infant diet in the first 6 to 12 months of life, with the rationale that early exposure to food allergens results in early sensitization, which leads to the development of food allergy.

There is evidence that the fetus has the capability of making immune responses and, specifically, IgE responses to milk and egg proteins as well as to some environmental allergens. This has led to the idea that restricting the mother's diet during pregnancy will lead to less food allergen exposure and therefore a lower risk of sensitizing the fetus, hopefully resulting in less food allergy for the baby. Several studies have examined the effect of avoiding milk and eggs during pregnancy on the development of food allergies and allergic disease in infancy. These studies, however, showed no benefit in preventing milk and egg allergy. A randomized prospective study by Robert Zeiger, M.D., also showed no benefit of maternal avoidance of milk, egg, or peanut during pregnancy in preventing allergies to milk, egg, and peanut through age seven.

In spite of these findings, however, the British Medical Council in 1998 recommended the avoidance of peanuts and peanut products by all pregnant and nursing women with newborns at high risk for allergies. These potentially allergic babies had either personal or family histories of allergies, asthma, or eczema. This recommendation may have been influenced the 1997 study by Jonathan O. Hourihane, M.D., which showed a relationship between increased maternal consumption of peanuts during pregnancy and lactation and earlier onset of peanut allergy in infancy and childhood. However, other studies examining the frequency of peanut allergy in children born to mothers eating peanuts during pregnancy have not confirmed this finding.

In 2009, a British study analyzed six previous studies of maternal pregnancy diet and early infant diet on the development of peanut allergy and found no relationship. However, the most recent study, in 2010, by Scott H. Sicherer, M.D., examined infants with eczema, milk, or egg allergy (infants considered to be at high risk for developing peanut allergy) and tested their sIgE to peanut. There was a significant correlation between the maternal consumption of peanut during the third trimester and the child having a positive sIgE to peanut. Although these infants had never eaten peanuts, it was felt that based on their peanut sIgE test level, they were likely to have allergic reactions if they did eat peanut.

Given the disparity of results in these multiple studies, the American Academy of Pediatrics stated in 2008 that there is no good evidence that dietary restriction during pregnancy will prevent the development of food allergies in children. The British Medical Council and various European medical organizations have issued similar statements since. The current guidelines for management of food allergies published by the National Institutes of Allergic and Infectious Diseases in 2010 also support these statements.

Is breast-feeding helpful in preventing food allergies?

Ellen's first baby was bottle-fed with infant formula. He was colicky in the first two weeks and needed several formula changes until he got better on a soy formula. At age two months, he developed eczema at about the same time foods were added to his diet. He was diagnosed with milk, egg, and peanut allergy by the pediatrician with positive RAST tests at age six months. He wheezed for the first time at age ten months when he had viral bronchiolitis. Since that time, he has wheezed with colds and respiratory infections. He is now three and wheezes with active play and running. His pediatrician feels that he has asthma. Ellen is pregnant with her second child and asks whether breast-feeding this baby will help prevent what her son has to go through.

Breast-feeding for the first six months of life is recommended by most pediatricians and the American Academy of Pediatrics. Human breast milk is nutritionally complete and contains everything the newborn and infant needs to grow and develop. Breast milk also contains numerous components of the immune system that help the baby defend against infection. These include protective antibodies that increase natural immunity and various enzymes that can kill bacteria, in addition to other protective elements of the immune system. Because of these benefits, all babies should be nursed, regardless of their risk for allergic disease.

As mentioned in the previous section, strategies of preventing the development of food allergies in genetically at-risk infants have focused on the possible benefits of exclusive breast-feeding. When the diets of these infants were studied, there seemed to be less eczema in the infants who were breast-fed compared to those who were fed milk formula. There is one study showing an association between exclusive breast-feeding for at least four months and decreased milk allergy but no benefit for decreasing allergies to other foods. Other clinical studies on exclusive breast-feeding do not show a protective effect on the development of food allergies in general.

Multiple studies have also been done on maternal avoidance of highly allergenic foods while breast-feeding; there was some benefit for decreasing eczema in the first 2 years of life, but no benefit for preventing food allergies from developing. Based on the current medical evidence, David M. Fleischer, M.D., and colleagues conclude that exclusive breast-feeding is recommended in at-risk children to reduce the development of eczema and milk allergy, but there would be no expected protection from developing food allergies in general.

Is hypoallergenic formula safer than breast milk?

Both breast milk and infant formula are nutritionally complete and equivalent in terms of nutrition and benefits for growth and development. Where breast milk has the advantage are the added components of natural antibodies and components of the immune system that protect the infant from infection. If breast-feeding is not possible, soy-based formulas and hypoallergenic formulas are available for infants with allergies to cow's milk. Hypoallergenic formulas are made by a process called hydrolysis in which the milk proteins are partially or extensively broken down, making them less allergenic. The extensively hydrolyzed formulas are less allergenic and recommended over the partial hydrolysate formulas for milk allergy. Good Start is a popular formula that is a partial hydrolysate formula. Nutramigen, Pregestimil, and Alimentum are extensively hydrolyzed formulas.

Can feeding with hypoallergenic formula prevent food allergies?

Using the same rationale as for breast-feeding, the question of whether feeding infants with hypoallergenic formula can prevent the development of food allergies has been studied. Fleischer and colleagues reviewed the medical literature on this topic and found that there was no advantage of feeding with hypoallergenic formulas over breast-feeding. Studies do show that for infants at risk for developing allergic disease who cannot be breast-fed for 4 to 6 months, feeding with hypoallergenic formula is beneficial in preventing allergic diseases and milk allergy. Extensively hydrolyzed formula was slightly more beneficial in preventing allergic disease; soy formula provided no benefit.

At what age should peanuts and tree nuts be introduced into a child's diet?

With the increasing prevalence of peanut allergy and reports of fatal and near-fatal anaphylaxis in the 1990s, there was much concern focused on the prevention of peanut allergy through dietary changes for the child. Based on the belief that the immune system of the gut in an infant is immature and susceptible to sensitization, especially with early exposure to highly allergenic foods such as peanuts and nuts, the American Academy of Pediatrics issued recommendations in 2000 for a schedule of introduction of solid foods to the infant genetically at risk for developing allergies. For allergenic foods, the recommendations were not to introduce milk until age one, egg at age two, and peanuts, nuts, and seafood at age three and older. These recommendations were somewhat arbitrary and not based on any evidence from clinical studies.

The hope was that delaying introduction of these foods responsible for the majority of childhood food allergies would stem the tide of the food allergy and peanut allergy epidemic. The opposite happened! Peanut allergy tripled in the United States from 1997 to 2008. Food allergies as a whole increased in the United States by 18 percent from 1997 to 2007. In the United Kingdom and Australia, where similar dietary guidelines were issued for delayed introduction of milk, egg, and peanut, the rates of food allergies dramatically increased as well.

Recognizing that the dietary guidelines issued in 2000 did not reduce food allergies, and acknowledging the lack of good scientific evidence for making the guidelines, the Academy rescinded those recommendations in 2008. European allergy organizations followed with similar retractions of their previous dietary guidelines. The problem remained, however, of how early these allergenic foods could be introduced into the baby's diet.

Is early introduction of peanuts and tree nuts into an infant's diet beneficial or harmful?

One interesting observation that would be useful in answering this question is the low prevalence of peanut allergy in many countries and regions of the world where, unlike the United States, United Kingdom, and Australia, peanuts are introduced early in the child's life, often in infancy. There is no peanut allergy epidemic occurring in Asia, Africa, and the Middle East where the infant diet seems to be the main difference.

However, it wasn't until a 2008 study by George DuToit, M.D., and his colleagues in the United Kingdom that scientific evidence indicated that delayed introduction of peanut in a child's diet might actually increase the risk of developing peanut allergy. This study examined 5,171 children in the United Kingdom and 5,615 Israeli children and found 1.85 percent of the British children had peanut allergy while only 0.17 percent of the Israeli children did. There were no significant genetic or ethnic differences between the two groups as both were of Jewish ancestry. The major difference was dietary: the monthly consumption of peanut in the British children was 0 grams, compared to 7.1 grams for Israeli children. Furthermore, Israeli children start eating peanuts as early as four to six months of age, often in the form of a popular snack called Bamba (corn puffs with peanut butter).

A study by Christine L. M. Joseph, Ph.D., and colleagues in 2011 showed lower rates of milk, egg, and peanut allergy when these foods were introduced into the infant diet at age four months or younger. Other studies have shown that early introduction of milk, egg, and wheat decreases the risk of allergies to these foods.

In light of these most recent studies, there is now a paradigm shift in how we think about how food allergies develop. It now seems more likely that there is a critical window of time for the infants' developing immune system, when exposure to a food protein triggers a "tolerance response" rather than an "allergic response." If introduction of that food is delayed, the opportunity to develop tolerance to that food may be lost. This concept may explain why the prevalence of peanut allergy greatly increased in countries including the United States, where delayed introduction of peanut to age three was recommended, and not in countries where children continued to start eating peanut at an early age.

What are the LEAP and EAT studies and what questions about a child's diet will they answer?

The research group led by Gideon Lack, M.D., that performed the studies on peanut allergy in Jewish children in the United Kingdom and Israel decided to do a prospective randomized controlled study to specifically answer the question of when to introduce peanut into the child's diet.

Entitled LEAP (Learning Early about Peanut Allergy), the study began in late 2007 and finished in 2013. Researchers recruited 640 infants ages four to ten months with either eczema or egg allergy who would be at high risk for developing peanut allergy, but who did not have a known peanut allergy at the time of recruitment. The infants were randomly assigned to either delaying introduction of peanut into their diets, following the old pediatric guidelines, or starting to consume 6 grams of peanut three times per week, similar to the Israeli infant diet. These children would be followed until five years of age, at which point the rates of peanut allergy will be examined for each group, to conclude which diet is associated with the development of peanut allergy. With the final results of the LEAP study, the question of exactly when peanut should be introduced to a child's diet should finally be answered!

The EAT study is a similar prospective interventional effort by the same group of investigators as the LEAP study. EAT (Enquiring About Tolerance) is a study of 1,302 infants ages 3 months and older, who will be randomly assigned to either exclusive breast-feeding for six months, or breast-feeding plus eating milk, egg, wheat, peanut, sesame, and fish. These infants will be followed to age three, at which time the rates of food allergies will be determined for each group to see which diet is associated with food allergies. Unlike the LEAP study, the majority of the infants recruited for the EAT study are from the general population, without risk factors for allergic disease. The EAT study will answer the question of whether early introduction of allergenic foods in infancy results in tolerance or allergy to these foods.

What is a reasonable schedule for the introduction of foods into the diet of a potentially food-allergic infant?

There are presently no universal recommendations or policies regarding this question. Based on available information from studies, most allergists would recommend strict breast-feeding for at least 4 to 6 months. Nursing supplements or weaning can be done with hypoallergenic formulas such as Nutramigen, Pregestimil, or Alimentum. These products are available in most pharmacies and many supermarkets. Solids can be started at ages four to six months and begun with foods such as rice cereal, fruits, and vegetables. Individual foods should be added sequentially weekly or biweekly, one food at a time. That way, if a reaction did occur, it would be easier to document the specific food that caused it.

Until the EAT and LEAP studies are completed, we do not have conclusive medical evidence for recommending exactly when to introduce allergenic foods such as milk, egg, wheat, peanuts, nuts, sesame, and seafood to a child. None of the current guidelines or specialty organizations has formally issued any specific schedule for families to follow.

An article published by Fleischer et al. in 2013, they reiterated the recommendation for exclusive breastfeeding for 4 to 6 months, followed by adding single-ingredient foods thereafter, no faster than one new food every 3 to 5 days. They suggested starting with rice or oat cereal, yellow and orange vegetables such as carrots and squash, fruits, green vegetables, and then age-appropriate staged foods with meats. They recommended not starting with the highly allergenic foods until after the preceding foods were tolerated. Another recent article by Kirsi M. Jarvinen, M.D., Ph.D., and Fleischer suggested a similar schedule:

Diet for infants at risk for allergy	Comments
Breast-feeding	First 4 to 6 months of age.
Supplementation	Partial or extensively hydrolyzed formula for first 6 months if unable to breast-feed.
Introduction of solid foods at 4 to 6 months	Yellow and orange vegetables, green vegetables, fruits, baby cereals (rice, oat, and wheat), and meats. Advance foods as appropriate for feeding skills. Introduce individual foods sequentially, one food per week.
Introduction of highly allergenic foods	Dairy, egg, peanut, tree nuts, fish, and shellfish can be gradually introduced after less allergenic foods have been tolerated. Allergy consult if an allergic reaction or moderate to severe eczema occurs, or peanut-allergic sibling.

Source: Immunology and Allergy Clinics of North America, 2012. Adapted with permission from W. B. Saunders.

CHAPTER 8

THE FUTURE OF PEANUT ALLERGY TREATMENT

Can peanut allergy be treated with allergy shots?

Allergy shots, or allergen immunotherapy, have been in use for the treatment of hay fever and asthma since the early 1900s. This form of treatment works by inducing an immunity to the various environmental allergens, such as pollens, molds, dust mites, and animals, with regular monthly injections of the allergenic material in graded minute amounts over a period of 3 to 5 years. Since the 1970s, allergen immunotherapy has been successfully used in the treatment of insect-sting anaphylaxis from honeybees, yellow jackets, hornets, and wasps by the administration of minute amounts of insect venom over 5 years or more.

For patients meeting the selection criteria, the success rate of immunotherapy for hay fever is as high as 80 percent, with the possibility of long-term remission of symptoms. The success rate for venom immunotherapy is even higher, at 90 to 95 percent, effectively curing this potentially fatal allergy. Usually, the main side effects of immunotherapy are allergic reactions localized to the site of the injection, but occasionally systemic reactions such as hives, runny nose, cough, wheezing, and anaphylaxis do occur.

Immunotherapy for food allergy

The use of immunotherapy for food allergy was first reported by British physician John Freeman in 1930. He was able to desensitize a 7-year-old boy who had unstable asthma triggered by fish ingestion, as well as hives, angioedema (swelling), vomiting, and diarrhea with fish exposure. The patient lost both his fish allergic reactions and his skin test reactivity to fish. He was able to maintain his desensitized condition by eating fish and taking cod liver oil every day. There were almost no subsequent reports of treatment of food allergy with immunotherapy in the subsequent decades because the standard treatment for food allergy continues to be avoidance and an elimination diet.

In 1987, John Carlston, M.D., of Eastern Virginia Medical School, published on the successful treatment of two patients with food allergies with food immunotherapy. The first patient had peanut allergy with anaphylaxis, including allergic symptoms caused by inhalation of peanut odor. She was treated with injections of peanut extract, starting at a dose of 0.05 ml of a 1:100,000 weight per volume dose that was gradually increased 150-fold to a maintenance dose of 0.5 ml of a 1:2,000 dose. This maintenance dose is the equivalent of $1/10$th of a teaspoon of a solution made by mixing 1 gram of peanut in 2 liters (more than 2 quarts) of water. This is a minuscule amount of peanut! She had frequent allergic reactions to treatment, including wheezing, but she did lose her peanut sensitivity, and after a year of symptomless peanut exposures her immunotherapy was stopped. She continued to do well on follow-up one year later.

The second patient was a seafood restaurant worker whose asthma was exclusively triggered by her working environment. She was treated with a mixture of fish (cod, flounder, halibut, mackerel, and tuna) and shellfish (clam, crab, scallop, oyster, and shrimp). Her asthma improved greatly, allowing her to work without symptoms, and she was also able to eat shrimp without problem.

In 1992, Harold Nelson, M.D., and Donald Leung, M.D., Ph.D., and their colleagues at the National Jewish Hospital in Denver published a randomized placebo-controlled study of peanut immunotherapy in patients with a history of peanut allergy and anaphylaxis.

Eleven patients began the protocol, and eight patients reached maintenance immunotherapy. Of the four patients finishing the study, three patients received peanut immunotherapy and one received placebo. The three patients who received peanut immunotherapy had a significant decrease in symptoms on DBPCFC and a decrease in skin test reactivity to peanut. The placebo-treated patient had no change in either DBPCFC or skin test reactivity. Unfortunately, systemic reactions occurred at the very high rate of 13.3 percent, almost four times that of pollen immunotherapy. The systemic reactions were all mild to moderate; there were no anaphylactic reactions in the three patients. This study is the first to demonstrate in a well-controlled manner that traditional immunotherapy can be an effective treatment for food allergy and anaphylaxis, dispelling the old dogma that immunotherapy for food is ineffective.

Presently, immunotherapy for food is still considered experimental because of the high incidence of side-effects and the lack of larger, more extensive controlled studies documenting the safety of the treatment.

What is oral immunotherapy for food allergy?
Oral immunotherapy (OIT), or oral desensitization, uses the same principle as allergy shots in desensitizing the patient to his or her food allergies by giving the patient very small but increasing amounts of the allergen orally instead of by injection. As early as 1908, there was a report of successful treatment of a child with egg allergy with oral desensitization. Over the years, there have been multiple reports of patients with food allergies successfully treated with oral immunotherapy to a variety of foods including milk, egg, fish, hazelnut, and peanut.

Recent clinical trials of peanut OIT have drawn much attention. Typically, subjects in these trials undergo an initial escalation phase usually in the hospital where they are started on low doses of peanut protein (often peanut flour mixed in a vehicle such as applesauce) and quickly advanced to a dose of 50 mg. This is followed by a buildup phase at home where daily doses of peanut protein are more slowly increased by 25 mg every two weeks until a maintenance dose of 300 mg is reached. The maintenance dose is continued on a daily basis indefinitely to maintain the "desensitized state." On this maintenance treatment, depending on the study, patients have been able to tolerate from 5 grams to more than 8 grams of peanut protein, which would provide adequate protection against most accidental exposures to peanut in the environment.

What are the short-term and long-term risks of peanut oral immunotherapy?

In 2013, Hugh Sampson, M.D., reviewed the results from eight clinical trials of peanut oral immunotherapy and made several observations. Most subjects who underwent peanut OIT could eat significantly more peanut protein after 4 to 6 months of treatment. However, more than 90 percent of subjects experienced adverse reactions, mostly mild, and 15 percent of all subjects in these trials had to drop out because of significant and persistent allergic reactions. There were also a number of conditions that could result in "breakthrough" allergic reactions to eating peanuts. These included viral illnesses and fever, active asthma and allergy symptoms, taking the maintenance peanut dose during exercise or menstruation or on an empty stomach. There was also a concern that some subjects developed recurrent gastrointestinal symptoms that became chronic, and some patients developed long-term chronic inflammation of the esophagus (eosinophilic esophagitis).

Are the benefits of oral immunotherapy permanent?

A major problem with oral immunotherapy to peanut is that the maintenance dose of peanut has to be taken daily for an indefinite period of time or else the desensitization is lost and allergic reactions to peanut recur. The long-term ability to tolerate peanut requires the daily maintenance dose of peanut long term.

What changes in the immune system result from oral immunotherapy?

Someone who is desensitized to an allergen by oral immunotherapy requires an ongoing exposure to the allergen to maintain that desensitized state. The reason has to do with the immunologic changes that result from oral immunotherapy. The ongoing exposure to peanut induces the immune system to make IgG antibodies (see chapter 1) that block the allergic response. Without continuing daily exposure to peanut, the blocking IgG antibodies are not made and the allergic reactions breakthrough and desensitization is lost.

People who are not allergic to peanut are considered to be tolerant of peanut. This state of "tolerance" is different than the state of being desensitized. People who have achieved tolerance do not need a daily maintenance dose of the food allergen to maintain tolerance. The "tolerant immune system" is characterized by special regulatory T cells (see chapter 1) that trigger a tolerance response and/or suppress allergic responses. These regulatory T cells are not found in patients who are allergic or who are only desensitized. These T cells do not require the continued exposure to the food allergen to perform their function. None of the studies on oral immunotherapy to foods have shown that permanent tolerance to foods is achieved by this treatment.

The ideal goal of any long-term treatment for peanut allergy is to achieve tolerance to peanut. Unfortunately, current studies indicate that oral immunotherapy achieves desensitization only, not tolerance. Based on all these issues and the need for more investigation, oral immunotherapy is not quite ready as a treatment for peanut allergy at this time.

What is sublingual immunotherapy for peanut allergy?

Just as allergy injection immunotherapy has been in use for treatment of allergic rhinitis and asthma, sublingual immunotherapy has been similarly used for treating these allergic conditions as well. Instead of the allergy extract materials being injected into the skin (subcutaneously), the extracts are administered under the tongue (sublingually). The absorption of the allergen is excellent because of the large number of blood vessels in the tongue area.

One advantage of sublingual immunotherapy (SLIT) has been its safety compared to traditional subcutaneous immunotherapy (SCIT); the main side effects of SLIT are minor localized itching of the mouth whereas severe allergic reactions including wheezing and anaphylaxis can occur with SCIT. Given its safety, SLIT treatment for a variety of food allergies have been reported over the years to kiwi, hazelnut, milk, peach, and peanut.

In 2013, David Fleischer, M.D., and colleagues reported the first randomized double-blind, placebo-controlled multicenter trial of SLIT for peanut allergy. Of twenty subjects receiving peanut SLIT, 70 percent were able to raise their dose of tolerated peanut from 3.5 mg to 996 mg after 44 weeks of treatment. Side effects were confined to itching and discomfort in the mouth, tongue, and lips; one patient had mild anaphylaxis requiring treatment with Benadryl and EpiPen. Although these were all encouraging results, none of the responders to treatment were able to tolerate 5 grams of peanut, indicating that clinically relevant protection might not be achieved with just 44 weeks of SLIT. In addition, responders to SLIT are likely to be desensitized only, and not immunologically tolerant. Further longer term studies are needed to assess the long-term outcomes of SLIT for peanut allergy.

What is epicutaneous immunotherapy for peanut allergy?

Another route of delivering the allergen for treatment is placing a patch containing the allergen on the skin. This is called epicutaneous immunotherapy (EPIT). A small study of eighteen children published in 2010 examined EPIT for milk allergy. Patches containing 1 mg of dried milk powder were placed on the skin for 48 hours at a time, three times a week for 3 months. After 3 months of EPIT treatment, the tolerated dose of milk increased from 1.8 ml to 23.6 ml, a clinically significant improvement, while the placebo treated group had no change. Common side effects to the patch were localized itching, redness, and eczema where the patch was applied. Based on these results, a clinical trial for peanut EPIT was begun in 2012; as of this writing, the trial was still in the recruitment stage.

Is Chinese herbal medicine helpful in treating food allergy?

Xu Min Li, M.D., and her colleagues at Mt. Sinai Medical Center in New York have studied the effectiveness of Chinese herbal medicines in preventing peanut anaphylaxis in peanut-allergic mice. The Chinese have used herbal medicines for centuries to treat of a variety of diseases, including allergies and asthma. Li purified the crude herbal mixtures and applied the treatment to her peanut-allergic mice. Mice sensitized to peanuts were treated with a formula of eleven traditional Chinese herbs named FAHF (for food allergy herbal formula) twice daily for 7 weeks. The mice treated with placebo herbs all developed anaphylaxis when challenged with peanuts while none of the mice treated with the herbal formula had any allergic symptoms for as long as 5 weeks following completion of treatment. The treated mice had lower levels of peanut-specific IgE, suggesting a possible mechanism of action for the herbs. There were no observed side effects in the treated mice.

Li subsequently refined the formula to nine herbs and with the new formula called FAHF-2 was able to completely block anaphylaxis to peanut in the peanut allergic mice. Li found that only brief treatment with FAHF-2 provided prolonged protection from allergic reactions to peanut, more than 5 months after the last dose of FAHF-2, suggesting that the mice had developed tolerance to peanut.

Li subsequently conducted a clinical trial in human subjects and showed that FAHF-2 was well tolerated with no significant side effects. The investigators found immunologic changes in regulatory T cells that seemed to mediate tolerance. A follow-up clinical trial with FAHF-2 is currently underway, studying patients ages 12 to 45 who are allergic to peanut, tree nuts, sesame seed, or seafood. Based on the immunologic changes observed in the mouse studies and human trial, it is thought that FAHF-2 may induce tolerance for allergic reactions to all foods, not just specifically for peanut. This novel approach is the first to induce tolerance rather than just desensitization. FAHF-2 has the potential to be the "cure" for food allergies we have all been searching for!

What does the future hold for the treatment of peanut allergy?

There are many exciting areas of research in food allergy. Better understanding of the immunology of allergic reactions as well as progress being made in the identification and characterization of peanut allergens with gene sequencing may one day make it possible to manipulate the immune response to these allergens. Once this becomes possible, it might be possible to "turn off" the allergic response.

One approach is to decrease the amount of circulating IgE in the patient. Antibodies to IgE can be made, which will bind to and remove IgE from circulation. Because the presence of IgE is required for all allergic reactions, this theoretically could be the answer to all types of allergic diseases, from food allergies to hay fever to eczema to asthma. These anti-IgE antibodies have already been studied in mice with good results, and several human trials in patients with hay fever and asthma show promising early results.

In 2003, Leung, Nelson, and Sampson's group in New York published a multicenter study examining the effects of anti-IgE injections in eighty-one patients ages 13 to 59 years with severe peanut allergy and histories of anaphylaxis. On average, these patients could not eat more than half a peanut before experiencing allergic reactions and anaphylaxis. After receiving injections of the anti-IgE vaccine for 3 months, they were able to tolerate up to nine peanuts without reacting at all. This type of treatment may be able to prevent the common types of accidental exposures occurring in restaurants and in cross-contaminated foods and reduce the frequency of anaphylaxis.

Although the original anti-IgE vaccine reported in 2003 is no longer available, Xolair, a similar anti-IgE vaccine available for the treatment of moderate to severe asthma, was subsequently studied by the same investigators in 2011. Treatment with Xolair resulted in 44 percent of subjects tolerating 1,000 mg or more of peanut flour, compared with only 20 percent of placebo-treated subjects. A 2012 study of Xolair treatment for peanut allergy showed that after 6 months of treatment, the quantity of peanut tolerated by subjects increased from the equivalent of one peanut to twenty-one peanuts. Current trials are studying the combination of OIT with Xolair. Dale Umetsu, M.D., and colleagues recently published a study showing the effectiveness of milk OIT combined with Xolair. There are now ongoing studies combining OIT with Xolair for peanut allergy.

Another novel approach to treatment is a DNA vaccine, which contains the DNA coding for peanut allergen Ara h 2. Injection of this DNA induces a suppressive immune response that "turns off" the response to Ara h 2, thus preventing any allergic reaction to peanut. This approach successfully reduced peanut anaphylaxis in mice and may potentially be applied to humans in the near future.

The main drawback to traditional immunotherapy with peanut extracts is the very high rate of allergic reactions both local and systemic to each injection. There is certainly a risk of anaphylaxis as well if an incorrect dose or error is made in the administration. To counteract this problem, the immunotherapy material can use peanut protein that has been modified to contain only the portion that is recognized by the patient's immune system (called **epitope**) but that lacks the portion that will bind to IgE on mast cells. In this fashion, the immune system will be able to generate the same type of immunity to peanut while, at the same time, not develop an allergic reaction to the injections because the allergen would be incapable of binding to mast cells. This type of immunotherapy has been called

peptide therapy because only the relevant portion of the whole peanut protein, called the peptide, is administered in the injection. Peptide immunotherapy has already been successfully studied in human trials with cat allergen and ragweed pollen allergen, and hopefully peanut peptide immunotherapy will tested in the future.

Using the principles of the hygiene hypothesis, which theorizes that the immune system turns "allergic" because it has not been stimulated with enough bacterial infections, scientists working with animal models have actually tried to "turn off" allergic immune systems with bacterial proteins. Some scientists have found that when using certain heat-killed bacteria combined with modified peanut proteins, peanut anaphylaxis could be prevented in peanut-allergic mice. Xu Min Li, M.D., and her colleagues have found success administering this combination as a rectal preparation in mice. They have subsequently started a phase-one clinical trial in humans using these heat-killed bacterial preparations.

Another approach using the principles of the hygiene hypothesis is to have allergic individuals take probiotics, which are "good bacteria." Probiotics are sold without prescription, such as lactobacillus acidophilus found in yogurt, lactobacillus GG, and bifidobacteria. They are commonly used to treat diarrhea caused by antibiotic use, generally considered safe, and are classified as supplements, not pharmaceuticals. Studies have shown that probiotics were able to reduce symptoms in shrimp-allergic mice. There are ongoing human studies examining the effectiveness of probiotics in preventing eczema and other allergic diseases such as asthma and hay fever and some evidence to show that there may be a benefit for reducing eczema. Probiotics have not been studied for peanut allergy. So far, there is no evidence in humans that food allergies are specifically prevented by using probiotics. You may wish to consult your doctor about this approach to dealing with allergies.

Perhaps the most interesting observation from the hygiene hypothesis is the protective effect of parasitic infections against asthmatic lung inflammation in experimental mouse models as well as several observational studies in humans showing reduction of asthma and allergies with parasitic infections. Using this rationale, a study by Mohamed E. H. Bashir and colleagues in 2002 showed that peanut-allergic mice infected with parasite had diminished peanut-specific IgE and anaphylactic symptoms were significantly decreased compared to noninfected peanut-allergic mice. Another study by Cathryn Nagler-Anderson, Ph.D., and colleagues in 2006 showed that having a parasite infection prevented the mice from being sensitized to peanut allergen.

Interestingly, the potential benefit of parasitic infection for other autoimmune diseases associated with the hygiene hypothesis is being investigated in inflammatory bowel diseases such as Crohn's disease, ulcerative colitis, as well as multiple sclerosis. Human studies in those diseases have already begun using the eggs of the whipworm, which normally infects pigs and generally do not infect humans. Safety studies in humans with whipworm eggs show no invasive infection and no significant clinical problems except for some patients having mild, transient gastrointestinal discomfort and diarrhea. The U.S. Food and Drug Administration has approved continuation of these clinical trials with whipworm.

A study led by Marie-Helene Jouvin, M.D., and colleagues examining the safety and possible protective effect of whipworm infection for peanut and tree nut allergy in humans has been approved at the Beth Israel Deaconess and Brigham and Women's hospitals in Boston. The study has begun recruitment of peanut- and tree nut–allergic adults ages 18 to 64.

A different approach to the problem of food allergy is to make the food itself nonallergenic, or hypoallergenic, through genetic engineering. Characterization of the three peanut allergens ara h 1, ara h 2, and ara h 3 has identified the portions of peanut protein that bind to IgE. It is this binding of the peanut allergens to IgE that triggers the mast cells to release histamine and the other chemical mediators causing allergic symptoms and anaphylaxis. Without binding of IgE to the peanut allergens, no allergic reaction would occur. Because the genetic structure and sequence of the three peanut allergens is known, scientists are now able to alter the peanut proteins and render them incapable of binding to IgE. Through genetic engineering, a new type of peanut could be grown, containing these altered proteins; these peanuts would not trigger any allergic reactions in peanut-allergic patients. Genetically engineered plants have already been available for years now, with qualities such as resistance to pests and disease, enhanced nutritional content, longer shelf life, and many other desirable features. The technology now exists for to greatly reduce the allergenicity of foods and to make them safe for all to eat.

Preliminary studies by Hortense Dodo, Ph.D., and coworkers show successful transformation of Georgia green peanut varieties with a modified ara h 2 protein. They are now growing these genetically modified hypoallergenic peanut plants to maturity and seed formation and will eventually be able to test these new peanut strains for their allergenic activity.

WHERE CAN I LEARN MORE ABOUT FOOD ALLERGIES?

The best single source of information on food allergies in general are your local allergy specialists. They have the special training to help clarify your various symptoms and make the diagnosis of specific allergies. Most importantly, they can give specific recommendations on allergy-control measures and avoidance strategies and give you the most current treatment based on the newest advances in allergy and immunology research. They will work with your primary care doctor in formulating a well thought out plan for managing your food allergies.

For the best resource available to the public on food allergies, the Food Allergy Research & Education (FARE), formerly FAAN, is unparalleled. They are a nonprofit organization that serves

> "to increase public awareness about food allergies and anaphylaxis, to provide education, and to advance research on behalf of all those affected by food allergies."

The organization was founded by Anne Muñoz-Furlong, whose daughter was diagnosed with milk and egg allergies as an infant. Lack of information and support for people and families with food allergies prompted her to form this organization, which is now not only the best resource for patients and families, but which is also involved in funding and conducting research and educational programs. It is active in the food and restaurant industry and in government and legislative issues. FAAN formed the National Registry of Peanut and Tree Nut Allergy for all peanut- and nut-allergic people to register and provide information about their allergy history. It now has a National Registry of Shellfish Allergy as well. These registries provide a valuable database, from which a number of important medical studies have already originated.

In November 2012, FAAN merged with the Food Allergy Initiative (FAI), a private foundation formed in 1998 to fund research in food allergy. The new organization is Food Allergy Research & Education or FARE. FARE continues the mission of FAAN with education and patient advocacy and the mission of FAI, to fund research that will increase knowledge and understanding of food allergy causes and eventually lead to treatments and a cure.

The website of FARE is the same as FAAN: www.foodallergy. org. The website is the most valuable resource for anyone with any food allergies. There are sections on education from which you can download the Food Allergy Action Plan and other school and camp forms, management guidelines, brochures for school staff, etc. There is a section on advocacy that has updates of the group's legislative efforts, state guidelines for schools, airline peanut policies, etc. You can also subscribe to allergy alerts for up-to-date information on food products, industry alerts, and changes in labeling.

FARE publishes a bimonthly newsletter, *Food Allergy News*, for adults and a separate one for children. They have many publications on specific topics, including peanut allergy, tree nut allergy, and understanding food labels. They have a useful cookbook, and recipes are included in every newsletter. They have excellent school programs as well as instructional videotapes, including one I highly recommend, *Alexander, The Elephant Who Couldn't Eat Peanuts*. One of the most useful services to patients is their Special Allergy

Alert Notices, which keep the public up to date on the food industry's latest news bulletins, product recalls, and warnings. I recommend FARE to all my patients with food allergies.

Other sources of information on food allergies or allergic diseases in general are the Allergy and Asthma Foundation of America (AAFA), the American Academy of Allergy, Asthma and Immunology (AAAAI), and the American College of Allergy, Asthma, and Immunology (ACAAI). AAFA provides educational programs to the general public and local support groups for patients and families with asthma and allergic diseases, including food allergies.

AAAAI and ACAAI are professional organizations for allergy and asthma specialists, but they do provide information and educational materials to the general public on asthma and all allergic diseases. They also have a referral directory so that patients can be given names of allergy and asthma specialists in their local communities. Both organizations have websites and can be found at www.aaaai.org and www.acaai.org, respectively.

WHAT ARE THE MAIN TAKE-HOME POINTS TO REMEMBER ABOUT PEANUT ALLERGY?

- Peanuts are one of the main causes of food allergies and, together with tree nut allergies, they are the leading cause of fatal and near-fatal food anaphylaxis.
- The prevalence of peanut allergy has tripled from 1997 to 2008.
- Most people do not outgrow peanut allergy (only 20 percent), unlike most other food allergies. Of those who do outgrow peanut allergy, 9 percent can relapse and become allergic again.
- The symptoms of allergic reactions include itching, hives; swelling of the face, throat, and tongue; abdominal pain, vomiting, diarrhea, difficulty breathing, wheezing, dizziness, loss of consciousness, and shock.
- Anaphylaxis is a systemic reaction that can lead to cardiovascular collapse and death. It requires immediate treatment with epinephrine.
- Anaphylaxis from food is almost always from ingestion or oral/mucosal contact and not from exposure to skin or inhalation.
- Because there is no cure as yet for peanut allergy, strict avoidance is the key to management.
- Accidental ingestions are a fact of life; 25 percent of peanut-allergic patients experienced accidental ingestions and reactions in the preceding year.

- Be prepared to deal with accidental ingestion and anaphylaxis when eating and traveling outside the home. Peanut-allergic individuals should have epinephrine (EpiPen, AuVi-Q, or Adrenaclick) on them wherever contact with food is expected, especially outside the home. They should also have a rapid-acting liquid antihistamine such as diphenhydramine (Benadryl).
- You should create a written emergency action plan (EAP) with your physician, keeping a copy for yourself and filing another with the medical office at the workplace or nurse's office in school. Children should also have a written individual healthcare plan (IHP) on file with their school, detailing preventive management in the classroom, cafeteria, on school activities and trips, on the school bus, and at all other locations that the child might be in.
- Conventional cleaning techniques are highly effective in removal of food allergen.
- Learn to read labels and ingredient lists.
- Be aware of the problem of hidden allergens, cross-contamination, and indirect exposures.
- When eating outside the home, inform people of your allergy, especially food servers, restaurant staff, school cafeteria staff, airline staff, and so forth.
- Peanut oil may not be safe if it has been contaminated through cooking or if it is crude, cold pressed, or unrefined.
- Peanut allergy is caused by a specific immunologic response to peanut protein.
- Peanut allergy is usually genetically determined and inherited.
- Peanut allergy is more common in an individual who has other allergic diseases such as hay fever, asthma, or eczema, and is more common in close relatives such as siblings, parents, and other relatives who have allergic diseases.
- Parents with allergic diseases will have children at higher risk of developing allergic disease, including food allergy.

- Confirm the allergy by consulting with an allergist who can evaluate the problem with allergy testing.
- The gold standard for the diagnosis of food allergy is the double-blinded placebo-controlled food challenge.
- Potentially allergic infants should be breast-fed for the first four to six months of life.
- There is no evidence that avoidance of allergenic foods during pregnancy or early childhood prevents or delays the development of food allergies. Recent research has actually shown the opposite—that early introduction of allergenic foods including peanut may actually reduce the risk of food allergies. Completion of the current dietary interventional trials (LEAP, EAT) will give some definitive evidence for more specific recommendations.
- The current research on potential treatments for food allergy, including peanut allergy, is very promising. Various types of desensitization, including oral, sublingual, and epicutaneous; anti-IgE treatment; and Chinese herbal formula are treatments under current human trials. Until then, education, increasing public awareness, and prevention remain the principal approaches to this increasingly common problem.

GLOSSARY

Allergen A substance that causes an allergy; in the case of food, this is usually a protein.

Allergic rhinitis An allergic condition characterized by nasal congestion, itching, sneezing, and mucous, usually caused by environmental allergens. Commonly called "hay fever," which is a misnomer because patients don't get fever and the allergen is not hay!

Allergy An abnormally high sensitivity to certain substances such as food, pollen, medications, or bee stings.

Anaphylaxis A severe, rapidly progressive, potentially fatal systemic allergic reaction characterized by hives, swelling, difficulty breathing, wheezing, and gastrointestinal symptoms.

Anaphylactic shock is characterized by a drop in blood pressure in addition to the aforementioned symptoms and is life threatening.

Angioedema Swelling of tissue. When angioedema occurs in a critical area, such as the throat or tongue, obstruction of breathing can result in a life-threatening reaction.

Antibody A protein produced in response to foreign substances such as bacteria, toxins, and **allergens**. Antibodies are essential elements of the immune system in the response to infection as well as allergic reactions. The antibodies that neutralize bacteria and viruses are IgG and IgM. The antibody produced in allergic reactions is **IgE**.

Antihistamine A drug that counteracts the effects of **histamine** by binding to **histamine receptors** on tissues. This makes it important in treating allergies of all types because histamine causes the symptoms of allergic reactions.

Ara h 1, 2, and 3 Three component peanut proteins that are more commonly associated with allergic reactions to peanut. **Ara h 5, 8, and 9** are component proteins that cross-reaction with pollen and other plant proteins and are not associated with allergic and anaphylactic reactions to peanut. See **Component Resolved Diagnostic test**.

Atopic dermatitis The medical term for **eczema**.

Asthma A chronic inflammatory condition of the lungs, resulting in difficulty breathing, coughing, chest tightness, and wheezing. It is commonly triggered by infection, allergy, and physical factors such as exercise and cold air temperature.

B Cell A white blood cell that produces antibodies such as **IgE**.

Bronchospasm Spasms of the airways in the lung causing obstruction resulting in the symptoms of **asthma**.

Casein A white, tasteless, odorless milk protein. It is the basis of cheese and is also used to make adhesives, plastics, and paint. The sIgE blood test to casein is predictive of whether a milk-allergic person can tolerate eating baked goods containing milk.

Component Resolved Diagnostic (CRD) test A new blood test that measures component proteins of foods. Research is showing that some component proteins of foods are more associated with allergic reactions than other components. For example, Ara h 2 is the component of peanut proteins, most likely to be associated with allergic reactions to peanut.

Conglutin One of the allergenic peanut proteins.

Cross-reaction The reaction between an allergen and IgE generated against a different, but similar, allergen, often belonging to the same family or category. For example, a person who is allergic to walnuts and experiences anaphylaxis to pecans has had a cross-reaction between walnuts and pecans.

Double-blind placebo-controlled food challenge (DBPCFC) The "gold standard" for diagnosing food allergy. In this procedure, neither the person tested nor the doctor (double blind) will know whether the placebo or the actual food is given. This procedure eliminates any bias factor from the study.

Eczema A chronic inflammatory skin condition, often associated with allergic triggers such as food or environmental allergens. It is more common in people and their relatives who also have asthma and allergic rhinitis.

Elemental A prepared, nutritionally complete **hypoallergenic** diet consisting of basic nutrients such as amino acids, fatty acids, and simple sugars and containing no allergenic proteins. It is in liquid form and available for infants, children, and adults.

Elimination A diet that has strictly and completely eliminated the specific food(s) you are allergic to. Children who follow an elimination diet are more likely to outgrow their food allergy.

Epinephrine The drug of choice for anaphylaxis, which relieves the skin, cardiovascular, gastrointestinal, and respiratory symptoms of an acute allergic reaction. EpiPen, Auvi-Q, and Adreniclick automatic injectors of the drug epinephrine are used to treat anaphylaxis.

Epitope The part of the food protein that is recognized by the immune system and targeted by antibodies such as IgE.

Gluten is the main allergenic protein in wheat and is also found in rye and barley.

Glycinin is one of the allergenic peanut proteins.

Glycoprotein Any protein containing a carbohydrate sugar component. Most allergenic proteins are glycoproteins.

Histamine A physiologically active chemical released by **mast cells** as part of the allergic reaction. Histamine causes all the symptoms of allergy such as itching, sneezing, swelling, mucous production, and wheezing. The actions of histamine are blocked by **antihistamine** medications.

Hydrolysate The product of hydrolysis, a chemical reaction that breaks down and degrades a chemical or food, such as soy or milk hydrolysate. Hydrolysates are not necessarily less allergenic than the parent compound.

Hypoallergenic Having a decreased potential to cause allergic reactions.

IgE The antibody produced by B cells that recognizes allergens. **Mast cells** attached to IgE will bind to specific allergens, which will result in the release of **histamine**. The resulting effects of histamine on the body are what we recognize as allergic symptoms.

Immunology The study of the structure and function of the immune system.

Immunosuppression Suppression of the immune system by drugs, radiation, or diseases such as malignancies and AIDS. When the immune system is suppressed, it no longer performs many of its functions such as recognizing self from nonself and fighting bacteria and viruses.

Intolerance An adverse reaction to food that is not mediated by the immune system. In gastrointestinal intolerances, it is because of an inability to digest certain foods, for example, lactose intolerance.

Lactalbumin is one of the **whey** proteins in milk.

Lactoglobulin is the other whey milk protein.

Mast The cell of the immune system that produces histamine and other chemical mediators involved in allergic reactions. **IgE**

attached to mast cells will bind allergen, causing the mast cell to release **histamine**. Mast cells are found in all the target organs of allergic symptoms, such as the skin, eyes, mucous membranes of the nose, sinuses, ears, lungs, blood vessels, and gastrointestinal tract.

Mediators Chemicals made by cells of the immune system that *mediate* various reactions in the body such as allergic reactions.

Oral Immunotherapy (OIT) A new treatment for food allergies in which the food-allergic patient undergoes a medically supervised protocol and receives very small measured amounts of the allergy-causing food, with subsequent increasing doses until a maintenance daily dosing schedule is reached. See chapter 8.

Ovalbumin is an egg-white protein.

Ovomucoid is another egg-white protein. The sIgE blood test to ovomucoid is predictive of whether an egg-allergic person can tolerate eating baked goods containing egg.

Peptide therapy A form of allergy therapy that involves injections of only the active allergic component (peptide) of the allergic protein. The theoretical advantage of this form of allergy injection is that there are much fewer allergic reactions and side effects to the injections.

Placebo A substance that contains no active ingredient as does a food or drug. It is used in medical studies as a control for patients who believe they are being given the active ingredient.

RAST (see specific IgE, sIgE) RadioAllergoSorbent test is a blood test used in the past to measure the level of **allergen**-specific **IgE** in your blood to determine whether you are allergic to that allergen. The term RAST is considered obsolete and has been replaced by the term **specific IgE**. RAST is still sometimes used generically (like Xerox for photocopy) for any allergy blood test.

Receptor A molecular structure or site on the surface of a cell that is able to bind to chemicals, such as **histamine**, or to proteins, such as antibodies like **IgE**.

Skin prick tests Skin tests are performed by pricking a pointed instrument or device through a drop of allergenic extract that has been placed on your skin. The skin is not broken; the prick enables enough fluid extract to penetrate the first layer of the skin. An allergic skin reaction comparable to a small mosquito bite will form if you are allergic to that allergen. Skin prick tests are a reliable way to diagnose allergies.

Specific IgE (sIgE) is a blood test that measures the level of allergen-specific IgE in your blood to determine whether you are allergic to that allergen. It is no longer performed by the old RAST method; it is now performed by the ImmunoCAP assay, so it is sometimes referred to as the ImmunoCAP test.

T cells The white blood cells that regulate immune function. T cells can direct the immune pathway to either allergy or tolerance.

Tolerance The state of being able to eat the food without allergic reactions. Tolerance can be natural, which is the normal condition of most people. Tolerance can be naturally acquired, such as an infant with milk allergy who outgrows it, or tolerance can be induced by some of the new treatments discussed in chapter 8.

Tropomyosin A muscle protein that is the main allergen in shellfish.

Urticaria The medical term for **hives**: a skin rash characterized by very itchy red welts usually caused by exposure to an allergen.

Vicilin is an allergenic peanut protein.

Whey is the watery part of milk that separates from the curds (also known as **casein**) when milk curdles. Whey contains **lactalbumin** and **lactoglobulin**.

APPENDIX D

REFERENCES

The references I have cited throughout this book are listed below for the more ambitious of you who wish to go to the primary sources. In addition to the following sources, *Food Allergy News* (FAN) the newsletter of Food Allergy Research & Education (FARE), is an invaluable reference source. There is also available from FARE a compilation of all the peanut allergy articles previously published in that newsletter.

American Academy of Pediatrics Committee on Nutrition. "Hypoallergenic infant formulas." *Pediatrics* 2000; 106:346–9.

Bernhisel-Broadbent, J., and Sampson, H. "Cross-allergenicity in the legume botanical family in children with food hypersensitivity." *Journal of Allergy and Clinical Immunology* 1989; 83:435–40.

Bock, S.A., et al. "Double-blind, placebo-controlled food challenge (DBPCFC) as an office procedure: A manual." *Journal of Allergy and Clinical Immunology* 1988; 82:986–97.

Bock, S.A. "The natural history of food sensitivity." *Journal of Allergy and Clinical Immunology* 1982; 69:173–7.

Bock, S.A. "The natural history of peanut allergy." *Journal of Allergy and Clinical Immunology* 1989; 83:900–4.

Bock, S.A., et al. "Fatalities due to anaphylactic reactions to foods." *Journal of Allergy and Clinical Immunology* 2001; 107:191–3.

Boyce, J.A., et al. "Guidelines for the diagnosis and management of food allergy in the United States: Report of the NIAID-sponsored expert panel." *Journal of Allergy and Clinical Immunology* 2010; 126:S1–S58.

Brown, S.G.A. "Clinical features and severity grading of anaphylaxis." *Journal of Allergy and Clinical Immunology* 2004; 114:371–6.

Buford, J.D., and Gern, J.E. "The hygiene hypothesis revisited." *Immunology and Allergy Clinics of North America* 2005; 25:247–62.

Burks, W., et al. "Peanut allergens." *Allergy* 1998; 53:725–30.

Carlston, J.A. "Injection immunotherapy trial in inhalant food allergy." *Annals of Allergy, Asthma & Immunology* 1988; 61:80–2.

de Montis, G., et al. "Sensitisation to peanut and vitamin D oily preparations." *The Lancet* 1993; 341:1411.

Dodo, H., et al. "A genetic engineering strategy to eliminate peanut allergy." *Current Allergy and Asthma Reports* 2005; 5:67–73.

Ewan, P. "Clinical study of peanut and nut allergy in 62 consecutive patients: New features and associations." *BMJ* 1996; 312:1074–8.

Ewan, P. "Prevention of peanut allergy." *The Lancet* 1998; 352:4–5.

Fleischer, D.M., et al. "The natural progression of peanut allergy: Resolution and the possibility of recurrence." *Journal of Allergy and Clinical Immunology* 2003; 112:183–9.

Fleischer, D.M., et al. "Peanut allergy: Recurrence and its management." *Journal of Allergy and Clinical Immunology* 2004; 114:1195–201.

Fleischer, D.M., et al. "The natural history of tree nut allergy." *Journal of Allergy and Clinical Immunology* 2005; 116:1087–93.

Fleischer, D.M., et al. "Primary prevention of allergic disease through nutritional interventions." *Journal of Allergy and Clinical Immunology: In Practice* 2013; 1:29–36.

Fleischer, D.M., et al. "Sublingual immunotherapy for peanut allergy: A randomized, double-blind, placebo-controlled multicenter trial." *Journal of Allergy and Clinical Immunology* 2013; 131:119–27.

Food Anaphylaxis Task Force of Massachusetts. *Managing Life-Threatening Food Allergies in Schools.* Malden, MA 2002. Massachusetts Department of Education. www.doe.mass.edu/cnp.

Fries, J. "Peanuts: Allergic and other untoward reactions." *Annals of Allergy, Asthma & Immunology* 1982; 48:220–6.

Goetz, D.W., et al. "Cross-reactivity among edible nuts: Double immunodiffusion, crossed immunoelectrophoresis and human specific IgE serologic surveys." *Annals of Allergy, Asthma & Immunology* 2005; 95:45–52.

Greer, F.R., et al. "Effects of early nutritional interventions on the development of atopic disease in infants and children: The role of maternal dietary restriction, breastfeeding, timing of introduction of complementary foods, and hydrolyzed formulas." *Pediatrics* 2008; 121:183–91.

Hefle, S.L., et al. "Consumer attitudes and risks associated with packaged foods having advisory labeling regarding the presence of peanuts." *Journal of Allergy and Clinical Immunology* 2007; 120.171–6.

Hourihane, J. "Peanut allergy—current status and future challenges." *Clinical & Experimental Allergy* 1997; 27:1240–6.

Hourihane, J. "Peanut allergy: recent advances and unresolved issues." *Journal of the Royal Society of Medicine* 1997; 30(suppl):40–4.

Hourihane, J., et al. "An evaluation of the sensitivity of subjects with peanut allergy to very low doses of peanut protein: A randomized, double-blind, placebo-controlled food challenge study." *Journal of Allergy and Clinical Immunology* 1997; 100:596–600.

Hourihane, J., et al. "Peanut allergy in relation to heredity, maternal diet, and other atopic diseases; results of a questionnaire survey, skin prick testing, and food challenges." *BMJ* 1996; 313:518–21.

Hourihane, J., et al. "Randomised, double blind, crossover challenge study of allergenicity of peanut oils in subjects allergic to peanuts." *BMJ* 1997; 314:1084–8.

Hourihane, J., et al. "Resolution of peanut allergy: Case-control study." *BMJ* 1998; 316:1271–5.

Hourihane, J., et al. "Resolution of peanut allergy following bone marrow transplantation for primary immunodeficiency." *Allergy* 2005; 60:536–7.

James, J. "Airline snack foods: Tension in the peanut gallery." *Journal of Allergy and Clinical Immunology* 1999; 104:25–7.

Jarvinen, K.M., and Fleischer, D.M. "Can we prevent food allergy by manipulating the timing of food exposure?" *Immunology and Allergy Clinics of North America* 2012; 32:51–65.

Johnson, M.J., and Barnes, C.S. "Airborne concentrations of peanut protein." *Allergy and Asthma Proceedings* 2013; 34:59–64.

Jones, R.T., et al. (abstract). "Recovery of peanut allergens from ventilation filters of commercial airliners." *Journal of Allergy and Clinical Immunology* 1996; 97:423.

Jouvin, M., and Kinet, J. "*Trichuris suis* ova: Testing a helminth-based therapy as an extension of the hygiene hypothesis." *Journal of Allergy and Clinical Immunology* 2012; 130:3–10.

Kelso, J.M. (Letter). "A second dose of epinephrine for anaphylaxis: How often needed and how to carry." *Journal of Allergy and Clinical Immunology* 2006; 117:464–5.

Klemola, T., et al. "Feeding a soy formula to children with cow's milk allergy: The development of immunoglobulin E-mediated allergy to soy and peanuts." *Pediatric Allergy and Immunology* 2005; 16:641–6.

Koerner, C., and Hays, T. "Nutrition basics in food allergy." *Immunology and Allergy Clinics of North America* 1999; 19:583–603.

Korenblat, K., et al. "A retrospective study of epinephrine administration for anaphylaxis: How many doses are needed?" *Allergy and Asthma Proceedings* 1999; 20;383–6.

Lack, G., et al. "Factors associated with the development of peanut allergy in childhood." *New England Journal of Medicine* 2003; 348:977–85.

Legendre, C., et al. "Transfer of symptomatic peanut allergy to the recipient of a combined liver-and-kidney transplant." *New England Journal of Medicine* 1997; 337:822–3.

Lehrer, S., et al. "Immunotherapy for food hypersensitivity." *Immunology and Allergy Clinics of North America* 1999; 19:563–81.

Leung, D., et al. "Effect of anti IgE therapy in patients with severe peanut allergy." *New England Journal of Medicine* 2003; 348:986–93.

Li, X., "Beyond allergen avoidance: Update on developing therapies for peanut allergy." *Current Opinion in Allergy and Clinical Immunology* 2005; 5:287–92.

Lieberman, J.A., et al. "Quality of life in food allergy." *Current Opinion in Allergy and Clinical Immunology* 2011; 11:236–42.

Lieberman, J.A., et al. "Bullying among pediatric patients with food allergy." *Annals of Allergy, Asthma & Immunology* 2010; 105:282–6.

Lieberman, P. "Biphasic anaphylactic reactions." *Annals of Allergy, Asthma & Immunology* 2005; 95:217–26.

Loza, C., and Brostoff, J. "Peanut allergy." *Clinical and Experimental Allergy* 1995; 25:493–502.

Maloney, J.M., et al. "Peanut allergen exposure through saliva: Assessment and interventions to reduce exposure." *Journal of Allergy and Clinical Immunology* 2006; 118:719–24.

McIntyre, C.L., et al. "Administration of epinephrine for life-threatening allergic reactions in school settings." *Pediatrics* 2005; 116:1134–40.

Monks, H., et al. "How do teenagers manage their food allergies?" *Clinical and Experimental Allergy* 2010; 40:1533–40.

Mulherin, K. "Day care center sued for discriminating against food-allergic children." *Food Allergy News* 1997; 6(3):3.

Muñoz-Furlong, A. "Food labeling rules, practices and changes to come." *Food Allergy News* 1996; 5:3.

Muñoz-Furlong, A. "Daily coping strategies for patients and their families." *Pediatrics* 2003; 111:1654–61.

Muñoz-Furlong, A. "Food allergy in schools: Concerns for allergist, pediatricians, parents and school staff." *Annals of Allergy, Asthma & Immunology* 2004; 93 (suppl 3):S47–S50.

Nowak-Wegrzyn, A., and Sampson, H.A. "Food allergy therapy." *Immunology and Allergy Clinics of North America* 2004; 24:705–25.

Nowak-Wegrzyn, A., and Sampson, H.A. "Future therapies for food allergy." *Journal of Allergy and Clinical Immunology* 2011; 127:558–73.

Oppenheimer, J., et al. "Treatment of peanut allergy with rush immunotherapy." *Journal of Allergy and Clinical Immunology* 1992; 90:256–62.

Perry, T.T., et al. "Distribution of peanut allergen in the environment." *Journal of Allergy and Clinical Immunology* 2004; 113:973–6.

Plaut, M. "New directions in food allergy research." *Journal of Allergy and Clinical Immunology* 1997; 100:7–10.

Rawas-Qalaji, M.M., et al. "Sublingual epinephrine tablets versus intramuscular injection of epinephrine: Dose equivalence for potential treatment of anaphylaxis." *Journal of Allergy and Clinical Immunology* 2006; 117:398–403.

Rix, K., et al. "A psychiatric study of patients with supposed food allergy." *The British Journal of Psychiatry* 1984; 145:121–6.

Rosen, J., et al. "Skin testing with natural foods in patients suspected of having food allergies: Is it a necessity?" *Journal of Allergy and Clinical Immunology* 1994; 93:1068–70.

Sampson, H. "Food allergy. Part 1: Immunopathogenesis and clinical disorders." *Journal of Allergy and Clinical Immunology* 1999; 103:717–28.

Sampson, H. "Food allergy. Part 2: Diagnosis and management." *Journal of Allergy and Clinical Immunology* 1999; 103:981–9.

Sampson, H. "Food allergy and the role of immunotherapy" *Journal of Allergy and Clinical Immunology* 1992; 90:151–2.

Sampson, H., et al. "Fatal and near-fatal anaphylactic reactions to food in children and adolescents." *New England Journal of Medicine* 1992; 327:380–4.

Sampson, H. "Managing peanut allergy." *BMJ* 1996; 312:1050–1.

Sampson, H. "Peanut allergy." *New England Journal of Medicine* 2002; 346:1294–9.

Sampson, H., et al. "Second symposium on the definition and management of anaphylaxis: Summary report—Second National Institute of Allergy and Infectious Disease/Food Allergy & Anaphylaxis Network symposium." *Journal of Allergy and Clinical Immunology* 2006; 117:391–7.

Sampson, H.A. "Peanut oral immunotherapy: Is it ready for clinical practice?" *Journal of Allergy and Clinical Immunology: In Practice* 2013; 1:15–21.

Shemesh, E., et al. "Child and parental reports of bullying in a consecutive sample of children with food allergy." *Pediatrics* 2013; 131:e10–17.

Shreffler, W.G., et al. "Microarray immunoassay: Association of clinical history, in vitro IgE function, and heterogeneity of allergenic peanut epitopes." *Journal of Allergy and Clinical Immunology* 2004; 113:776–82.

Sicherer, S., et al. "Clinical features of acute allergic reactions to peanut and tree nuts in children." *Pediatrics* 1998; 102(1). www.pediatrics.org/cgi/content/full/102/1/e6.

Sicherer, S., et al. "Genetics of peanut allergy: A twin study." *Journal of Allergy and Clinical Immunology* 2000; 106:53–6.

Sicherer, S., et al. "Prevalence of peanut and tree nut allergy in the U.S. determined by a random digit dial telephone survey." *Journal of Allergy and Clinical Immunology* 1999; 103:559–62.

Sicherer, S., et al. "Prevalence of peanut and tree nut allergy in the United States determined by means of a random digit dial telephone survey: A 5-year follow-up study." *Journal of Allergy and Clinical Immunology* 2003; 112:1203–7.

Sicherer, S., et al. "Self-reported allergic reactions to peanut on commercial airliners." *Journal of Allergy and Clinical Immunology* 1999; 103:186–9.

Sicherer, S. "Clinical update on peanut allergy." *Annals of Allergy, Asthma & Immunology* 2002; 88:350–61.

Sicherer, S., and Sampson, H. "Food allergy." *Journal of Allergy and Clinical Immunology* 2006; S470–5.

Sicherer, S.H., et al. "U.S. prevalence of self-reported peanut, tree nuts and sesame allergy: 11-year followup." *Journal of Allergy and Clinical Immunology* 2010; 125:1322–6.

Sicherer, S.H., et al. "Maternal consumption of peanut during pregnancy is associated with peanut sensitization in atopic infants." *Journal of Allergy and Clinical Immunology* 2010; 126:1191–7.

Simons, E., et al. "Can epinephrine inhalations be substituted for epinephrine injections in children at risk for systemic anaphylaxis?" *Pediatrics* 2000; 106:1040–4.

Simons, E., et al. "Epinephrine for the out-of-hospital (first aid) treatment of anaphylaxis in infants: Is the ampule/syringe/needle method practical?" *Journal of Allergy and Clinical Immunology* 2001; 108:1040–4.

Simonte, S.J., et al. "Relevance of casual contact with peanut butter in children with peanut allergy." *Journal of Allergy and Clinical Immunology* 2003; 112:180–2.

Skolnick, H.S., et al. "The natural history of peanut allergy." *Journal of Allergy and Clinical Immunology* 2001; 107:367–74.

Smith, A.F. "Peanuts: The illustrious history of the goober pea." University of Illinois Press, Chicago, 2002.

Smolowe, J., and Lambert, P. "Kiss of Death," *People*, December 19, 2005. pp. 116–22.

Steinman, H. "Hidden allergens in foods." *Journal of Allergy and Clinical Immunology* 1996; 98:241–50.

Teuber, S., et al. "Allergenicity of gourmet nut oils processed by different methods." *Journal of Allergy and Clinical Immunology* 1997; 99:502–7.

Vadas, P., et al. "Detection of peanut allergens in breast milk." *Journal of the American Medical Association* 2001; 285:1746–8.

Wang, J., and Li, X.M. "Chinese herbal therapy for the treatment of food allergy." *Current Allergy and Asthma Reports* 2012; 12:332–8.

Webb, L., et al. (abstract) "Anaphylaxis: a review of 593 cases." *Journal of Allergy and Clinical Immunology* 2004; 113:S240.

Weeks, R. "Peanut oil in medications." *The Lancet* 1996; 348: 759–60.

Wensing, M., et al. "The distribution of individual threshold doses eliciting allergic reactions in a population with peanut allergy." *Journal of Allergy and Clinical Immunology* 2002; 110:915–20.

Wood, R. "More answers to commonly asked questions about anaphylaxis." *Food Allergy News* 1999; 8:6.

Young, M.C., et al. "Management of food allergies in schools: A perspective for allergists." *Journal of Allergy and Clinical Immunology* 2009; 124:175–82.

Yunginger, J. "Lethal food allergy in children." *New England Journal of Medicine* 1992; 327:421–2.

Yunginger, J., et al. "Fatal food-induced anaphylaxis." *Journal of the American Medical Association* 1988; 260:1450–2.

Zeiger, R. "Prevention of food allergy in infants and children." *Immunology and Allergy Clinics of North America* 1999; 19:619–46.

INDEX